'Jennifer Harper's *Nine Ways to Body Wisdom* is a readable and re[...] and Natural Medicine. I recommend it whole-heartedly.'

Peter D'Adamo, ND, Author, *Eat Right fo[...]*

'*Nine Ways to Body Wisdom* is a perfect title for this accessible work that distils the insights of ancient Chinese Medicine and the wisdom of the body into a wonderfully practical handbook. It brings a wealth of information to everyone, whether a beginner or a seasoned practitioner.'

Donna Eden, Author, *Energy Medicine*

'Whilst the popularity of complementary therapy has increased enormously in recent years, the orthodox profession is only now beginning to express a grudging respect for many of its benefits – particularly for disorders which conventional doctors find unsatisfactory to treat. Jennifer opens our eyes to a whole new therapeutic universe and she does it clearly, methodically and most important of all, responsibly.'

Dr Hilary Jones, GP, and Author, *The Complete Encyclopaedia of Natural Medicine and GMTV doctor*

'This book skilfully integrates the ancient art of Chinese Medicine with contemporary nutritional science in a highly practical and user-friendly way.'

Patrick Holford, Author, *Optimum Nutrition Bible*

'A goldmine of easy to read information for those who want to take more responsibility for their health.'

Hazel Courtenay, *Sunday Times,* and Author, *What's the Alternative?*

'A book that should be read by doctors, therapists and those interested in complementary therapies, to give them a further understanding of a holistic approach to healing, using Jennifer's clear and well presented explanations.'

Matthew Manning, Healer, and Author, *One Foot in the Stars*

'Despite being a practitioner of homoeopathy and complementary therapies for the last 25 years I have always found it difficult to have an intuitive gut feeling for Chinese Medicine, possibly because I have been so steeped in the Western paradigm in my medical education. Jennifer Harper's book has come as a refreshing change to the usual text on Chinese Medicine. She has explained it in very down-to-earth terms and has managed to combine it with other complementary therapies such as reflexology, acupuncture, diet and exercise in an easy to follow manner. I would recommend it both for orthodox medical practitioners who wish to gain an insight into the Chinese way of thinking regarding health and also for other complementary therapists who are not practitioners of Chinese Medicine and who have difficulty relating to it.'

Dr Andrew Lockie, GP, Homoeopath, and Author, *The Family Guide to Homoeopathy*

'This is a book of balance, how to restore it, maintain it and use it for both prevention and treatment of illness. After 40 years of using Naturopathy, Acupuncture and Traditional Chinese Medicine I can safely say that Jennifer's book embraces the fundamental truths of natural positive health. Her clear concise style makes these sometimes complex philosophies accessible to all.'

Michael Van Straten, ND, Author, *Organic Superfoods*

'Jennifer Harper has taken the often confusing principles underlying Traditional Chinese Medicine and skilfully presented these in a way the Western mind can easily see the sense of. Her own gifts as a natural healer and her dedication to helping everyone discover the wisdom of their own body and its healing powers shines through on every page.'

Susan Clark, *Sunday Times,* and Author, *Vitality Cookbook*

'"Packages of care" are the coming thing. Increasingly we will see practitioners suggesting lifestyle changes and self-help tailored to their treatments. Jennifer's approach comes in a Chinese Medicine shaped package combining diet, exercise and inner-path instructions. For her, integration is clearly more than just bringing together unrelated ideas and practices, because her notions of energy and harmony make life-style changes meaningful. And meaning can motivate. I would heartily recommend her book to practitioners and patients with a feeling for the Dao.'

Dr David Peters, Clinical Director, University of Westminster, and Author, *The Encyclopedia of Complementary Medicine*

'This is a timely and remarkable text, bringing to life and making accessible the wisdom of Traditional Chinese Medicine. Jennifer has given everyone the chance of helping themselves towards better health by offering a truly holistic approach to healing – bringing together body and spirit.'

Leon Chaitow, ND, Author, *Antibiotic Crisis: Antibiotic Alternatives*

'Jennifer has courageously drawn together the ancient principles of Chinese Medicine with simple, practical, understandable Western techniques and treatments that can be used not only to help the body heal ailments but also to empower the person.'

Leslie Kenton, Author, *Journey to Freedom*

'Today Jennifer is trying to build bridges between orthodox medicine and alternative medicine to arrive at a complementary system which will help human suffering in more efficient ways. It is wonderful to see these coming together, not only because of the changes in medicine which have taken place but because people like Jennifer have put all their efforts into making the systems known and giving people the freedom of choice in the way they are treated. This book is an eye-opener on long-proven methods which will improve your health and happiness.'

Jan de Vries, ND, Author, *Inner Harmony*

# nine ways to body wisdom

*blending natural therapies to nourish
the body, emotions and soul*

Jennifer Harper ND PhD MSc

Thorsons

Thorsons
An Imprint of HarperCollins*Publishers*
77-85 Fulham Palace Road,
Hammersmith, London W6 8JB

The Thorsons website address is www.thorsons.com.

Published by Thorsons 1997, 2000
10 9 8 7 6 5 4 3 2 1

A catalogue record for this book is
available from the British Library

The diagrams on pages 256 and 258 are
based on originals by Pierre J. Cousin

ISBN 0 7225 3368 3

Printed and bound in Great Britain by
Woolnough Bookbinding, Irthlingborough, Northants.

*To my parents and Celia with love*

# the author

Jennifer Harper is a qualified naturopathic doctor and herbalist who has
an MSc in Complementary Therapies and a PhD in Natural Health. She
is a gifted healer and Reiki Master who runs her own clinic where she
believes in treating the 'whole' person by using a combination of natural
therapies including nutrition, Western and Chinese herbs, acupressure,
applied kinesiology, reflexology, therapeutic massage, aromatherapy and
flower remedies. With over ten years of postgraduate study, her Body
Wisdom Healing Programme has benefited numerous patients over the
years by providing a system that helps re-balance the body and achieve
optimum levels of health and wellbeing.

Jennifer is an inspirational speaker and has researched and presented
many different aspects of alternative medicine for television and radio.
She writes health-related features for a variety of top magazines and
offers natural health advice in monthly columns. Her media work is
focused on helping people more clearly understand the body and what
its symptoms and emotional states represent according to both Eastern
and Western medicine. Jennifer Harper's simple message demystifies the

abstract concepts found in Chinese medicine and various other alternative therapies that are suitable for self-healing, making the wisdom of these practices more accessible to the public.

# acknowledgements

Without the constant love and support on all levels of my parents, Tom and Mary Harper, I would not have been able to dedicate the amount of time necessary to really perfect *Nine Ways to Body Wisdom* and give the book the true attention that the concept deserves. Staying on the personal front, I would like to thank three special women in my life, Celia, Alexandra and Maggie, who are there to listen, support, guide and encourage me through all my ventures, both personal and professional – thank you for your patience, belief and vision. To my brother Simon and his lovely wife Tanya, thanks for watching over your little sis and ensuring that I take needed 'time-outs' from my work, and to Sue, Ruth, Vivienne, Stella, Tannis, Annie, J&J and JC. To Dana, my trusted and loyal house angel and Martin, my brilliant organic gardener who tends to my herbs, vegetables and flowers, thank you both for often going beyond the call of duty and helping me in so many ways. To Ivy and Jim thank you for walking and looking after my beautiful Weimerana dogs, Lola and Angel, when meetings take me away from them. Cuddles to my adorable dogs and to my other Rescue animal, my healing kitty Balloo

Bear, you remind me to laugh and play when life becomes too hectic. And to Clay, my partner in crime, without you my love, this new edition would not have come into reality. Thank you from the bottom of my heart for your tolerance and understanding of my commitment and dedication in helping others find their own wisdom within. It is my personal quest and my life's work to offer guidance and healing to people – I thank you for joining me on this journey.

To Stephen at Solgar, thank you for the genuine interest you have shown in the work I do in providing accurate nutritional information to the public. Add me to the list of people who have benefited from your knowledge, passion and clear focus. To Marie at Solgar, what a pure spirit you are – thank you for your constant support of my educational projects – as an educator working alone, certain business relationships stand out from others and it is important I thank you not only for your support but for your friendship as well. To Wanda Whiteley, for being much more than my editor by believing in the good this book could do for others and allowing *Nine Ways to Body Wisdom* to be released as it is. To Diana Mossop, a special soul who is on a parallel mission to mine in helping others – your research, work and new understanding of flower essences' power to heal has taken flower remedies to the next level. Also my special thanks for offering your meridian formulas to me, which are now an essential part of my own remedies. To Monica Linford, another special soul who has taken the concept of the five elements into the fitness world and developed her own exciting Chi Ball Method. To Jennifer, George, Maryam and Sam at Aveda, thank you for believing in my mission as I believe in Aveda's all-organic mission to care for the world we live in and to set examples for environmental leadership and responsibility... how refreshing! To Clare and Maleka at Origins – thank you for spending your time and energy as well as lending an ear to my ongoing effort to educate the public on natural health and for being involved in a company that is committed to preserving the earth by protecting the animals and environment. To Ian at Savant/Udo's Choice, thank you for your genuine and valued support of our shared goal in raising the public's awareness of the importance of essential fatty acids in the diet. To Scott and Kim from Klamath Blue Green, Inc. in the US – I have for years preached the wonderful benefits of blue green algae and want to thank you for making the effort and investment years ago to foresee the need that would arise for consistent quality control in Blue Green Algae production. To Nancy and Andrew from the Really Healthy Co., thanks for introducing this wonderful blue green stuff to the people of the UK. To Colette and Elaine at *Here's Health* Magazine, thank you for giving me the opportunity and providing me with such a respected and popular magazine from which I can spread my message. To Charlotte and Sue at Green People and Gaye at Hambledon Herbs, thank you for your sincerity and openness – it's great to see such a worthwhile effort made by you in getting the message out to the public on the importance of high quality organic products. To Sebastian from Dr. Hauska, thank you for your support and for being involved with a new breed of company that recognizes the importance of providing natural products that not only address the body's physical needs, but place as much emphasis on spiritual needs as well. To my dear colleagues from the herbal world, P.J. and Vicky, thanks for your input and testing out the Body Wisdom Organics formulas. To Sanjay, the brainchild behind the innovative store, Farmacia, which integrates conventional pharmaceutical goods with natural products and services. I hope that this concept will become a model for more pharmacies in the future. And also to my photographer Keith from Goodness Gracious, thanks for working your magic by taking such a warm and natural cover photograph.

Finally, I would like to extend thanks to all my patients and those of you who have experienced the positive and life changing benefits that the Body Wisdom programme can have on your health and wellbeing. It further reinforces my belief in the power of natural healing and the wisdom to be found in many ancient methods of medicine.

# contents

# foreword

It is with the greatest pleasure that I write the foreword for a book which is not only very impressive but looks at health in general from a completely different angle to that of most health books. The writer has gone into deep research of different alternative methods of how one can help oneself to better health. Along with the possible conventional approaches, there is a lot that patients themselves can do to improve their health mentally, physically and emotionally. Complementary medicine is looking at man not having one body but three: unless there is harmony in the physical, mental and emotional bodies, there will always be trouble. This book shows ways to look at these three bodies as, in today's society, we often see more problems of the third body, the emotional body, which is very often neglected and also a mighty weapon in one's own hands if one knows the ways to approach it. Whatever treatments, alternative or conventional, there is no improvement unless one has a positive mind. Positive action, in whatever treatment, will be of utmost importance as there is no improvement in health unless patients are relaxed and in full harmony with themselves and the people treating them. It needs a lot of self-education to arrive at this point.

I have known Jenni for many years and, when she was still quite young I was surprised at the terrific hunger and thirst that she had to help others. She studied, kept asking and asking and, in so doing, became a very busy student, educating herself and looking at all kinds of methods of helping others. It is this sharing which is so important in life; Jenni tries not only in her writing and in her personal consultations but also in her radio and television interviews to share with others what she has learned, and also the methods which she has tried which have worked and helped patients.

Today Jenni is trying to build bridges between orthodox medicine and alternative medicine to arrive at a complementary system which will help human suffering in more efficient ways. Orthodox medicine is a result of the technical revolution and has not been with us for very long. Alternative medicine has been with us for as long as we can remember and is defined as the original medicine. With all aspects of the two systems, which I have been practising for over 35 years, I have come to the conclusion that while a very sophisticated medicine can be of help, a very simple, long-forgotten herb can sometimes do the job even better. It is wonderful to see that, in today's society, these systems are coming more and more together, not only because of the changes in medicine which have taken place but because people like Jenni have put all their efforts into making the systems known and giving people freedom of choice in the way they are treated.

This is where a book like Jenni's fills a gap. It combines alternative treatments with other methods which have been proven to be successful. It is important that not just the obvious symptoms are cured, as conventional medicine teaches us. We have to look for the cause of the illness and, in looking at the cause, we come to understand how much we can do ourselves, with diet and simple methods which can be applied when necessary.

We learn every day that we have lost contact with grassroot levels. We have to realize that we belong to nature, we have to obey the laws of nature and, in so doing, we obey the laws of our creator. I am quite sure that this book will be of great help to many and, as Jenni has put so much effort into this, it will also be an eye-opener on long-proven methods which will improve your health and happiness.

Jan de Vries

D. Ho. Med., D.O., M.R.O., H.D., M.R.N., D.Ac, M.B.Ac

# introduction

While putting the finishing touches to *Body Wisdom*, I met a cardiac surgeon from Vienna, Dr Kassal Hermann. We were discussing the importance of health and how it is so often neglected or taken for granted. He told me a wonderful Austrian quote, which translates as:

*Health is not everything, but without health everything is nothing.*

How many of us can say that we respect our bodies and value our health? Hippocrates, the Father of Medicine, appreciated the significance of good health when he said those famous words

*A wise man ought to realize that health is his most valuable possession.*

Stress and strain seem to go hand in hand with life in the 20th century. More than ever before, we need to search for ways to re-establish harmony and equilibrium in our mind, body and spirit; to find a better way of taking care of ourselves by listening to our bodies and becoming more in tune with them. Do we know what our body is trying to tell us with the symptoms that it is displaying? These symptoms are so important as they are early warning signs that nature shows us in the hope that we can take preventative measures. The wise soul takes heed of these and will try to find the cause of the problem, as this is where the solution will be found and where self-healing begins.

In *Nine Ways to Body Wisdom*, I outline my own holistic approach and philosophy which greatly assists the process of self-healing by rebalancing the body's major internal systems. The Traditional Western Understanding section of each chapter may feel like a human biology lesson back at school, but it is crucial that a connection is made between the health of your organs and the health of your body. This information, coupled with the interpretation and significance of each organ according to Traditional Chinese Medicine (TCM), will provide you with empowering knowledge about the importance of the inner organs of the body and what they can reveal, so that you will have a greater understanding of the wisdom that lies within.

When we seek to restore or build our levels of health, we gain the greatest results when working with a variety of healing methods which help to nourish and support weak organs and body systems. This book, therefore, includes a variety of 'holistic' methods (i.e. ones that balance the psychological, physical and spiritual levels) to help strengthen and create balance in the body. These methods acknowledge that the mind, body and spirit need to be treated as a living unity and are based on the fundamental belief that the individual plays a vital role in his or her own healing. The therapies are simple and highly effective and when combined with the wisdom of Chinese medicine, create an exciting new way of working with the body.

Incorporating the effective self-help measures outlined in my book can help you correct imbalances in their early stages – that is, before they develop into common illnesses.

> *A doctor who treats a disease after it has happened is a mediocre doctor ...*
> *a doctor who treats a disease before it happens is a superior doctor.*
> Yellow Emperor's Classic of Internal Medicine (ca. 2nd century BC)

Following the nutritional recommendations, practising the therapies and exercises for body and mind, will enhance your knowledge of how to stay well, prevent the onset of certain diseases and improve the quality of your life. Start to trust and develop your own intuition or instinct, while continuing to seek advice wherever it can be found: your GP's surgery, with a homoeopath, a healer, nutritionist, reflexologist, acupuncturist, aromatherapist, etc. or someone skilled in many aspects of natural healthcare; and with your own 'inner doctor', who knows what is best for you. Never underestimate the body's own healing mechanism: it is extremely powerful and can reverse and repair most of the body's disharmonies, given the right conditions.

I hope that you will find that the 9 Ways to Health outlined in each chapter will provide you not only with valuable information, but more importantly, give you simple, practical techniques and advice that you can begin to integrate into your daily schedule, no matter how busy that schedule may be. We can all take 5–10 minutes out of our day to stretch our meridians, breathe more efficiently, rub some oils into our body and reflex points, say some affirmations. In fact, I will often combine many of these techniques together and while stretching, apply some oil to an acupressure point and mentally repeat positive affirmations! Self-knowledge and personal changes of this nature take both time and patience, but by following this holistic approach, the effects will be more powerful and longer lasting as they take into account the close interrelationship between your mind, body and spirit. I hope that you will feel inspired to learn a great deal about yourself and experience the wonder and wisdom of Chinese and natural medicine. Your body is prepared to tell you what is going on with it, if you are prepared to listen, feel and observe. When you personally experience the benefits firsthand, you will want to make the *Nine Ways to Body Wisdom* a regular part of your daily routine and your life as you will feel restored and revitalized.

Jennifer Harper ND PhD MSc

# past and present

Hippocrates, the Father of Medicine, referred to a highly beneficial healing energy that flowed through all living things as the *vis medicatrix naturae* – the 'healing power of nature'. This is the foundation on which the majority of therapies that come under the heading of 'alternative' or 'complementary' medicine are based. Nature cure or naturopathy is a system of health-orientated medicine which recognizes that the body has an inherent ability to heal itself and is a way of life which advocates living according to natural principles. Twenty-five centuries ago, Hippocrates believed that patients could often heal themselves by employing proper procedures and thus they had considerable responsibility for their health.

> *Health is the expression of a harmonious balance between various components of man's nature, the environment and ways of life ... nature is the physician of disease.*
>
> Hippocrates

After Hippocrates, Galen was considered to be the most important advocate of healing, believing that every organ in the body was activated by it. Plato, a contemporary of Hippocrates, taught that man had the power to heal himself. He realized what has often been ignored with the advent of science, that man was a trinity and illness was due to an imbalance in the mind, body and spirit. Plato held that the physician should begin with man's mind and soul and criticised physicians for their single-mindedly materialistic approach to illness, complaining that the greatest travesty of the day was the way in which their practice separated the body from the soul. Hahnemann, the Father of Homoeopathy, also felt that the true nature of all healing was spiritual. True healing involves the healing of our physical, emotional, psychological and spiritual being, a view also shared in the East as the Indian, Japanese and Chinese cultures all hold the same conviction that healing cannot be addressed on a physical level alone, believing that man is a multi-dimensional being made up of mind, body and spirit.

In the 17th century, the Hippocratic doctrine was superseded by a new approach that was soon to embody the philosophy of modern medicine as we know it today. René Descartes introduced the 'analytical' model and because it was so radically different, ultimately the principles underlying modern medicine came to be referred to as 'Cartesian'. The Cartesian approach separated the mind from the body and consequently the work of natural physicians went into decline. Chemistry and analysis dominated thinking and medicine began its retreat away from nature. This new philosophy embodied the principle that if plants contained simple, effective compounds then why not make a synthetic version of the active ingredients and bypass nature altogether? The emphasis of medicine changed from supporting the body's power to heal itself by restoring balance to the mind, body and spirit to one where the body was reduced to structural parts such as organs, tissues and cells.

The physician in his new role was able to separate the whole into individual parts in an attempt to discern the function of each component; the offending 'diseased' component could therefore be isolated and removed by surgical intervention or treated by the use of medication. However, this restricted outlook has limited the scope and effectiveness of medicine as it has tended to equate the cure of disease with the control of symptoms. Perhaps here we should reflect on the wise words once spoken by the Greek philosopher Plato:

> *The cure of any part should not be attempted without treatment of the whole. No attempt should be made to cure the body without the soul and if the head and body are to be healthy you must begin by curing the mind, for this is the great error of our day in the treatment of the human body that physicians first separate the soul from the body.*

Today, however, we are experiencing a resurgence in the popularity of natural methods and holistic techniques where the aim is to restore and promote balance in the 'whole' person. Until relatively recently, it had been viewed that allopathic (orthodox) medicine was incompatible with 'alternative' therapies. However, we are swiftly moving towards finding a place where both sides can work together in a fully integrated system of healthcare. The World Health Organization's goal is 'health for all by the year 2000'. Perhaps in the twenty-first century we will create a system which recognizes that physical, bio-chemical, psychological, spiritual and environmental factors all play a part in governing the state of our health; a system which respects and accepts the diversity, individuality and potential of each human and where the ultimate aim is to restore equilibrium to all levels of our being and sustain it.

# chinese medicine:
# an introduction

Traditional Chinese medicine (TCM) is a system of diagnosis and health-care which has evolved over the last 4,000 years and is a unique approach to understanding the human body. In Chinese medicine, health is viewed as a complete state of wellbeing, which is a different approach to Western medicine, which defines health as merely the 'absence of disease'.

TCM is based on the belief that all humanity is part of the natural environment and that health or balance can only be achieved when one follows the natural law, adapting to the changes of the seasons and the surrounding environment. This is the philosophy of the *dao*, and the Chinese believed (and still do today) that the more we stray from living in harmony with the *dao*, the more certain it is that no form of external medicine or treatment could ever compensate for the stresses that will affect mind, body and spirit. The theories of *yin* and *yang*, together with the notion of the five elements, were developed through ancient Chinese rituals of observing nature's ever changing cycles. These theories are fundamental to Chinese medicine.

## the five elements

The five elements are Wood, Fire, Earth, Metal and Water. These are related to the different seasons of the year and to organs in the human body. By knowing and understanding these elements, we can discover how to balance the extremes of each season and comprehend what unique opportunities for growth arise with each. The organs are inter-linked with the seasons, temperatures, colours and tastes, to name but a few associations, all of which have some relevance to our health and well-being. The five element theory shows the interrelationship of the organs in a very general way. However, it is essential to understand that the relationships between the different organs can be very complex. Sometimes it may be that one element is out of balance, but when disease is chronic it is very likely that all of the key organs could be affected to a greater or lesser degree.

The Wood phase occurs in Spring, which is a time in nature of activity and new beginnings. This is followed by the Fire Element in Summer, which is the season of abundance where the ideas that were put into action in the Spring have blossomed and flowered. The Earth phase arrives in late Summer and is the harvest season, a time when we can reap the benefits of the seeds planted in the early Spring. Metal is connected with Autumn, the time of decline when nature slowly begins to withdraw in preparation for the Winter. The life force in nature lies dormant during the Winter months of the Water Element, like the latent seed that is lying still and waiting to burst open in the Spring to begin the cycle once again. (See table on *page 9*.)

## emotions

Today, Western medicine is at long last beginning to validate the healing power not only of the body, but of the mind. Exciting research has trans-formed our concept of the mind and it is now thought that the mind has a presence throughout the entire body. This is because the cells which carry emotions in the brain have recently been discovered to exist in our immune system. The Chinese have understood for thousands of years that our thoughts and emotions have a great impact on the state of our health and that emotional distress compromises the health of the body.

This is why emotions play an important role in this book and are discussed in each of the chapters on the organs. There are five emotions, which are connected to the five elements and to the major *yin* organs (the liver, heart, spleen, lungs and kidneys). Anger relates to the liver, joy to the heart, pensiveness to the spleen, grief to the lungs and fear to the kidneys. Extremes of emotions can have a negative impact on the organs, especially when they are intense or have been suppressed for some time, just as an imbalanced organ can have a profound effect on the state of our emotions.

## EARTH

Worry or sympathy are the emotions connected to the Earth Element. Sympathy can display itself at times when we are over-sympathetic to circumstances or, alternatively, cannot bear people fussing over us. Someone who continually seeks as much sympathy as possible, the individual who happily tells you all about their health problems and woes, or who is constantly worrying, has an imbalance in the spleen or stomach.

## WOOD

Excessive amounts of anger or feelings of frustration, irritation or suppressed rage point to the Wood Element and show us that it is not functioning harmoniously. The Chinese, however, readily admit there are appropriate times for expressing anger and it is better to vent our feelings rather than to seethe and suppress this powerful emotion.

### FIRE

Laughter and joy are valuable emotions and today there is sadly not enough of these wonderful emotions on display. Someone who can't laugh or show love and affection, or who demonstrates excess amounts, reveals a Fire imbalance.

### WATER

Fear is a very real emotion and without it we might not realize when we are in dangerous situations. It can, however, consume us and this is when it is damaging to the Water Element.

### METAL

Finally, grief too is an important emotion that we experience when we go through the loss of something special. If there is an imbalance in the Metal Element, the grieving process can be prolonged beyond its natural term.

## yin and yang

Traditional Chinese medicine holds that the material world is in a constant state of flux due to the movement of *yin* and *yang*, two opposing elements which are mutually dependent (that is, they cannot exist without one another). The theory of *yin* and *yang* is used to help explain the physiological imbalances and any pathological changes in the human body. The resulting information is then used for diagnostic purposes. All the major organs in the body are paired according to the principles of *yin* and *yang* and with one of the five elements.

# qi

*Qi* or *chi* (pronounced 'chee') can be translated as 'vital energy' or life-force, but even these words do not capture what *qi* really is. It has been described as the force that nourishes both the body and mind, and the free-flow of this vital energy around the body is seen as imperative to our health and wellbeing. If the *qi* becomes imbalanced, or there is a blockage (*stagnation*), there is too little (a *deficiency*) or even too much (*excess*), disease can result. The flow of this vital energy can be impeded by poor diet, lack of exercise, poor breathing and posture, scar tissue and psychological stress.

*Qi* flows through the body in pathways called *meridians*.

# the meridian system

The ancient Chinese philosophy of energy is referred to as the meridian system. The meridians are channels that carry the *qi* around the body. Diagrams dating back to 3000 BC have been discovered on walls of caves depicting the flow of energy through these meridians. This ancient system has been used for centuries to heal and treat a broad range of imbalances in the body. The meridian channels act rather like the circulatory system which ensures that the blood travels throughout your body and can be likened to an 'energy' bloodstream. Although in modern society we use more electrical technology than ever before, in the West we still remain suspicious and sceptical of the vital importance of free flowing energy through our bodies for health. Thus the importance of electrical or energetic medicine has never really been fully understood or respected. There are 12 major organ meridians and eight extra channels. Both acupuncture and acupressure work on specific points along the meridians called acupuncture points. If these are congested it can impede the energy flow, possibly resulting in pain or problems in the associated organ. Meridians are a useful means of detecting imbalances in the organs well in advance of more chronic problems developing. Working on chosen points on the meridian can help to redirect and circulate the energy to the organs that need it, thus establishing harmony in our system.

Phytobiophysics, developed by Dame Diana Mossop is a powerful new scientific philosophy designed to treat the complex health problems of modern society by utilizing the energetic properties of plants to restore the correct flow of energy through the meridian system of the human body. The fourteen Phytobiophysics Meridian Flower formulas have been compiled as a result of many years of alchemy and research into combining the different energies of plants and are designed to tune the meridians and restore optimum function. Our combined effort has produced a powerful range of potent remedies that draw on the strength of flower formulas as well as a range of flower essence blends by Body Wisdom Organics which combines specific Phytobiophysics meridian formulas to bring balance to each of the five elements. These powerful meridian flower essences are contained in an organic herbal or flower tincture to allow a resonance with the physical body and organs.

There are 12 major meridians, two which are not covered in detail in this book are the pericardium and triple warmer or triple energizer. These are not linked to physical organs in a sense but have very important roles to play in health. The pericardium, is known as the 'heart protector' whose key function is to stop anything harmful from reaching the heart. The triple warmer regulates the temperature of the internal organs and has a connection to our thyroid gland that ensures we have a healthy metabolism. The Phytobiophysics formula FF9 Bluebell is designed to support the triple energizer and thyroid and the two meridians are included in the Body Wisdom Organics Fire Element Flower Formula.

There are also eight Extra Meridians that include the Conception vessel (also known as the *yin* or central meridian) and the Governing vessel (or *yang* meridian) yet only these two are considered to be major meridians as they both have specific meridian points unlike the other six Extra Meridians. The Phytobiophysics formula FF1 activates the pineal master controller and supports the Governor vessel and FF2 is the formula for the Conception vessel.

## lifestyle

Our lifestyle and its effects on our health are very important factors in Chinese medicine, especially in the areas of diet, exercise and sexual activity. Diet is an important factor in most cultures and the Chinese are no different; Chinese diets are, in a sense, more holistic and primarily designed to heal many common ailments, from constipation and diarrhoea to colds or skin disorders. The Chinese approach is far more complete than the Western one, as it dates back to the time before foods were classified according to their protein, fat, carbohydrate and nutrient content. The Chinese focused on the different qualities and primary actions of foods which were used to help create balance in the body. This system is known as food energetics; according to this system, all foods have specific qualities and effects on the body.

Exercise is an important factor, but it is a matter of balance: moderate exercise gets the *qi* flowing in the body but excessive amounts drain our vital kidney energy and can weaken the body. Understanding the concepts of duality and of balancing rest with activity is essential. According to TCM, too much sex can weaken the body thus reducing our vitality and energy levels. This is explained in greater depth under the chapter on the Kidneys (*page 145*).

## body clock

Every organ in the body has a two-hour period of maximum activity which means that when the organ is in its natural time period, it has greater energy than the others. If we honoured these times and let them guide us in our activities we would be much healthier. If you find that you have a dip in energy or feel worse at a particular time of day, then this could be pointing to the particular organ which falls into that time period. For example, the stomach is in power between 7 and 9 a.m. This is the time that digestion is at its peak. Therefore, the old advice 'Breakfast like a

King, lunch like a Prince and dine like a Pauper' is in fact quite correct, as breakfast is the time of the day when the body digests foods best. If you feel particularly tired between 5 and 7 p.m. in the evening, your kidney energy may not be as strong as it should be. If you can't get to sleep between the hours of 11 p.m. and 3 a.m., then your Wood Element is out of balance and needs treatment.

## early signs of disease

The wonder of the Chinese system of medicine is that changes often begin to occur approximately six to nine months *before* a disease arises. We can pick up on the particular stress signals that nature is providing if we can understand more about the body and know what signs to look out for. The body can show imbalances in a variety of ways: a hatred or passion for a particular season of the year, a love of a particular colour or a desire to avoid wearing a specific colour, or even a change in the colour of your face. Your body will emit a specific odour when an organ becomes imbalanced, and your emotions will change (since the organs in the body influence our emotions). By understanding and listening to your body, you can find out why it is functioning the way it is and then take the necessary steps towards improving your health.

The table opposite charts the traditional Chinese interpretations given to each of the five elements and its related organs.

*For a more in-depth look at Chinese Medicine, see pages 253–273.*

# five elements table

| | Wood | Fire | Earth | Metal | Water |
|---|---|---|---|---|---|
| Direction | East | South | Centre | West | North |
| Colour | Green | Red | Yellow | White | Blue/Black |
| Climate | Wind | Heat | Humidity | Dryness | Cold |
| Season | Spring | Summer | Late Summer | Autumn | Winter |
| Yin Organ | Liver | Heart | Spleen | Lungs | Kidneys |
| Time | 1–3 a.m. | 11a.m.–1 p.m. | 9–11 a.m. | 3–5 a.m. | 5–7 p.m. |
| Yang Organ | Gall Bladder | Small Intestine | Stomach | Large Intestine | Bladder |
| Time | 11 p.m.–1 a.m. | 1–3 p.m. | 7–9 a.m. | 5–7a.m. | 3–5 p.m. |
| Stage | Birth | Growth | Transformation | Absorption | Storage |
| Number | 8 | 7 | 5 | 9 | 6 |
| Planet | Jupiter | Mars | Saturn | Venus | Mercury |
| Spirit | Hun | Shen | Yi | P'o | Zhi |
| Body Tissue | Tendons/ Ligaments | Blood Vessels | Muscles/Flesh | Skin | Bones/ Marrow |
| Voice Sound | Shouting | Laughter | Singing | Weeping | Moaning |
| Emotion | Anger | Joy | Worry/ Sympathy | Grief | Fear |
| Taste | Sour | Bitter | Sweet | Spicy | Salty |
| Odour | Rancid | Burnt | Fragrant | Pungent | Putrid |
| Sense Organ | Eyes | Tongue | Mouth | Nose | Ears |
| Reflector | Nails | Complexion | Lips | Body Hair | Head Hair |
| Secretion | Tears | Perspiration | Saliva | Nasal Discharge | Sputum |

**N.B.** The time for the *pericardium* is 7–9 p.m.; for the *triple warmer*, 9–11 p.m.

# the nine ways to body wisdom

## introducing the therapies

This section explains the background of the therapies included in the *Nine Ways to Body Wisdom*: what they are and how they work, together with general guidelines and information on relevant techniques.

I have chosen a cross-section of natural therapies that I combine in my own clinic as I believe that the greatest results are gained by working with a variety of healing techniques to nourish and support weak organs and body systems.

Please note that although I have separated the organs into individual chapters to make them easier to understand, it is important to remember that these organs and body systems are completely interconnected and must not be seen as isolated structures – they are part of the 'whole'.

# way 1: chinese and natural nutrition

## WHAT IS CHINESE NUTRITION?

Diet is important to most cultures and the Chinese traditional view on nutrition is no different. Food is considered to have very potent healing properties or energies. Diets are traditionally holistic and designed to heal many common ailments ranging from the common cold to skin disorders.

## HOW IT WORKS

Traditional Chinese Medicine teaches that certain foods and flavours act on the 10 internal organs; some foods have a positive effect on more than one organ. Carrot, for example, works on both the lungs and spleen; celery works on the stomach and kidneys. This basic relationship between the internal organs and flavours has been studied over many years; the Chinese tradition believes that a combination of five flavours ensures balance, harmony and vitality in the body. Foods also have different properties – for example, cool, warm, dry or damp – and too much of any one food can have adverse effects. For example, warming foods are considered to raise the metabolic rate and cooling foods to lower it… an interesting fact as most Western diet books focus on raw (cold) foods such as fruit and salads for weight loss!

**Pungent** foods act on the Metal Element. Examples include green onions, chives, cloves, parsley and coriander. Their main action is to induce perspiration and stimulate circulation.

**Sweet** foods act on the Earth Element. Examples include cherries, bananas, honey and watermelon. They slow down acute symptoms and neutralize the toxic effects of other foods.

**Sour** foods act on the Wood Element. They include lemons, rhubarb and plums. They can help with diarrhoea and excessive perspiration.

**Bitter** foods act on the Fire Element. Examples include seaweed, bitter lettuce, coffee, asparagus and kelp. They influence the heart and small intestine, can reduce body heat, eliminate excess body fluids and induce diarrhoea.

**Salty** foods act on the Water Element. They include salt, seaweed and kelp, and affect the kidneys and bladder.

### GENERAL DIETARY GUIDELINES

Choosing the correct foods and dietary programme will always be an individual matter, but there are various guidelines that can start you off on the right track.

1   Try to eat meals in the right frame of mind, in other words, do not sit down to a meal if you are feeling angry or frustrated. Being calm and relaxed while you eat is almost as important as the food you consume. A peaceful state of mind aids digestion and assimilation of all the nutrients in the foods you eat. Using all your senses when you eat the meal, such as smelling the food, visually enjoying the look of your meal and tasting it, means that the body will be far more prepared to absorb the food.

2   Chew your food properly, as starch digestion begins in the mouth. Chewing your food also means that you take more time to eat the meal and, therefore, the body will have time to tell you when it is getting full. Rushing food down, as is common practice in today's society, means that we do not recognize the 'full' sign until we have gone past it!

3   Cut down on coffee, tea, alcohol, fried/fatty foods, refined convenience products and sweets. Caffeine is a stimulant that inhibits the absorption of vitamins and minerals in the body, but if you really cannot do without a cup of tea or coffee in your day, at least choose a superior brand, ideally an organic version too.

introducing the therapies

4   Increase your consumption of water. If the weather is cold, make sure that the water you drink is slightly warmed (at least room temperature) rather than ice cold. Cold water can cause the stomach to contract.

5   Eat whatever grows locally, and according to the seasons. Nature has given us the ideal foods to cope with each temperature and season. Eating salads in Winter is not ideal (unless you have had a warming meal prior to this), just as you probably wouldn't choose to have carrot and turnip stew on a hot Summer's day! The current trend focuses on eating foods as raw as possible. However, in the Chinese tradition, too much raw or 'cold' food in the diet is known to extinguish the 'digestive fires'. Too much cold food may lead to a 'damp spleen', which can give rise to symptoms such as oedema, weight gain, loose stools and abdominal bloating.

6   Do not eat late in the evening. At this time the body is naturally going into a 'rest' phase and cannot digest food properly. It is far better to eat a good breakfast when the stomach is in power (between 7 and 9 a.m.) and digestion is at its peak.

7   Eat whole foods and organic produce where possible. Pesticides and chemicals used in modern farming practices are very harmful to the immune system and liver. If you have no choice, wash produce in either cider vinegar and water, or salt water. There are also manufactured products available from health shops which are designed to eliminate agricultural residues.

8   When cooking grains and pulses, soak them overnight in filtered water with a little vinegar and a piece of kombu seaweed. Discard the liquid and cook them in fresh water. This process will break down the compounds that can cause gas and also increase the nutritional value and digestibility of the food.

9   Avoid cooking with nonstick pans, aluminium and copper, as these materials can leach metals into the food. Stainless steel, glass or earthenware are better choices.

10  Avoid food that has been either genetically modified, irradiated or microwaved.

**nine ways to body wisdom**

**Foods**

米   There is a lot of new research coming out in the US which suggests that we are not eating sufficient protein due to an obsession with low-fat and high-carbohydrate diets. Ensure that you are getting enough good quality protein. Buy organic meats wherever possible and keep to lean cuts – and remember, fresh fish is always preferable to frozen. Also, avoid fish from very polluted waters. Seeds (*see below*) are a good source of non-meat proteins, as are organic soya-based products such as tofu.

米   Increase your consumption of vegetables, but not raw ones when you are first making changes to your normal diet. This is because raw foods are very good cleansers, and if the body is very toxic the cleansing reaction will be too powerful. It is best to start gently, so eat plenty of home-made vegetable soups, lightly steamed vegetables and stir-fries.

米   Stir-frying is an excellent way of cooking vegetables as the nutrients are sealed within and you can include wonderful fresh herbs such as garlic, ginger, coriander and fenugreek sprouts. It is best not to use oil, however, as fats when heated change chemically and are not very good for the liver. Instead, use a little boiling water, to start sweating garlic, onions and ginger. When these have released some moisture, add more spices and then finally your vegetables.

米   Sprouting sesame, pumpkin and sunflower seeds increases their nutritional value so they become real 'superfoods'. These three seeds combined produce protein, but remember to chew them particularly well to ensure that your body will utilize and assimilate them readily. Sprinkle onto porridge, soups, stir-fries, etc. Other foods to sprout include mung and aduki beans, alfalfa and chick peas. Leslie Kenton's books have a lot of information on sprouting and include useful tables illustrating the length of sprouting times for different seeds.

米   Cut down on acidic grains such as wheat and rye and start including more wholegrain brown rice, millet and quinoa in your diet. The latter two are excellent with millet being alkaline, rich in iron, magnesium and silica (so great for your hair too!) and able to help cleanse and lower acid levels in the body. Quinoa, the mother food of the Incas, supports the kidneys. It is very high in protein and nutrients including vitamins B and E and minerals including calcium and iron. All these are excellent cleansing foods, which are at the same time very gentle on the system.

※ Raw, cold-pressed virgin seed oils are an excellent addition to the diet and can be mixed into a fresh salad dressing, thus adding essential fatty acids to the diet. Essential fatty acids help to regulate every organ, cell, tissue and system in our entire body. For example, they benefit our skin, our hormones, support our endocrine system so often weakened by high stress levels, and strengthen our immune system. I use Udo's Choice oil which contains a blend of unrefined organic flaxseed, sunflower and sesame oils, providing a 2:1 ratio omega 3 to omega 6 essential fatty acids. Do remember to keep the oil refrigerated and you can freeze additional, unopened bottles to properly preserve the fatty acids.

I am a great believer in natural supplements and will always take fatty acids and green super foods such as the Klamath blue green algae throughout the year. The Living Organics Superfood Formula by Body Wisdom Organics is a single nutritional, energetically balanced organic supplement which I have developed to contain a complete range of vital nutrients such as natural vitamins, trace minerals, amino acids, enzymes and probiotics. These key nutrients are carefully preserved from living organic sources and are concentrated in a form that the body can assimilate easily and efficiently. Drawing from the wisdom of the Five Elements in Traditional Chinese Medicine (TCM), this advanced formula also contains the five key herbs and spices essential in strengthening specific body systems, thus balancing all five elements.

Living Organics Blue Green Energetics formula is an organic, wildcrafted whole food from one of the purest lakes in the sparsely populated North Western United States. This green food is harvested during the summer months and freeze-dried for optimum preservation of its nutrients. Ginger and cinnamon are added to energetically warm and balance the formula, thus providing support to vital organs such as the kidney and spleen. Strengthening these organs helps our body to restore and regenerate, increases our energy levels, improves our digestion and boosts our sexual *qi*. All the formulas by Body Wisdom Organics have been developed to synergistically complement each other and can be taken in combination to nourish and support the organs.

❉ Keep your saturated fat intake as low as you can: grill foods and follow the boiling water method of cooking outlined earlier.

❉ It is also best to avoid citrus fruits such as oranges as they are known as 'aggressive' cleansers, and if your liver is not as strong as it should be, it may experience difficulty breaking down the fruit acids. Oranges are known to increase mucus levels in the body. The Chinese believe that too much fruit in Winter is not to be recommended as it does not grow naturally at this time of the year.

❉ When the weather is warm, more salad foods can be included in your diet. In Winter, a small salad can be eaten at the end of your meal if desired. Use oils high in essential fatty acids or cold-pressed virgin olive oil mixed with apple cider vinegar to make up a dressing for the salad (include fresh garlic and herbs).

❉ Herb teas and drinks such as Caro, Barley Cup or Bambu can be consumed, but have them without cow's milk or sugar. If you are a tea drinker, try Chinese Green tea. This contains antioxidants and the caffeine levels are lower and far less concentrated than those found in black tea. However, it should still be consumed in moderation!

### Breakfast

❉ Breakfast could be oatmeal porridge, preferably using organic oats and apple juice or water, not milk, to moisten.

❋ Milk is difficult to digest and often contains hormones, steroids and antibiotics. Dairy foods increase the production of mucus in the body, and a large number of people cannot efficiently digest these foods. I consider the best alternatives to be almond milk, rice milk, oat milk, sheep and goat's milk.

### Lunch

❋ Lunch could consist of a home-made vegetable soup or brown rice with vegetables. If you follow a food combining programme (*see Suggested Reading, page 304*), then the above is fine, or if you want a protein meal, exchange the rice for a protein dish of your choice.

### Dinner

❋ Dinner could be a repeat of the above, or a stir-fry with fresh organic vegetables and either millet, rice or quinoa. Again, protein can be added to the meal. It is a good idea to soak any of the grains used for between 12 and 24 hours, as this increases their nutritional value and makes them easier to assimilate in the body. It is best to restrict your intake of puddings; if necessary, nibble on unsulphured dried fruit that has been soaked in mineral water for several hours.


## way 2: herbs and spices

Traditionally many common herbs and spices have been used by cultures throughout the world. In Egypt the temples actually had laboratories where both essential oils and plant medicines were produced. Folk law has many ancient recipes validating the healing power of herbal concoctions that have been passed down and perfected through the centuries. Traditional Chinese Medicine is one of the oldest healing arts and along with diet, exercise and acupuncture points, herbs too formed a major part of the therapeutic programme used by the Chinese to bring the body back to harmony and prevent illness. Like Galen, one of the forefathers of modern medicine, Chinese medicine categorized herbs 'energetically', that is, classified them as having such properties as cooling, heating, drying or moistening.

Plants have been extensively researched by the pharmaceutical industry, the active ingredients being isolated to produce drugs. Over seventy percent of the drugs in the British Pharmacopoeia have their origins from herbs. White willow bark is a natural analgesic (pain killer) and was used to form aspirin and digoxin from the foxglove became a popular heart drug. However, herbalism supports the notion of using the 'whole' plant as they believe that plants are complex and contain many synergistic ingredients within that work together to make the plant a potent form of natural medicine.

Herbal medicines are being used by an increasing number of the population as the public is looking for gentler forms of treatment. In the past, pharmaceutical drugs were assumed to be more effective than herbal remedies, but many studies now highlight that natural products are just as potent as modern medicines, but have the distinct advantage of causing fewer side effects providing they are used correctly. Mounting scientific evidence also supports the healing power of plants as researchers have been comparing both the safety and efficacy of natural remedies with their chemical counterparts. This has resulted in numerous scientific studies and research papers appearing in prestigious scientific journals worldwide, including the *Lancet* and the *British Medical Journal*.

There are several excellent ways to use herbs to heal your body including herbal teas, tinctures, dried herbs in capsule form and herbs that are applied externally (which includes essential oils). Herbs form the foundation of many formulas for many of the natural therapies that are popular today and it is hard to find a natural product that does not in some way draw on the power and therapeutic benefit of herbs. As part of my Body Wisdom programme, I have formulated a range of herbal products called Body Wisdom Organics, that are energetically balanced according to the particular needs of the organs and are based on years of studying Eastern and Western herbal medicine and patients responses to herbs. The essence and effectiveness of these products result from the appropriate combination of herbs in the formulas, as well as using potent, pure and all-organic herbs. Due to my commitment to the environment, this range uses only environmentally friendly packaging as well as special dark violet bottles that protect the potency of the product from light degradation.

As a practising herbalist, I have seen medicinal herbs successfully treat conditions where modern medicine has failed, so I have great faith in the power of plants. However, it is important to realize that there can be dangers in self-prescribing and if you have any doubts at all, before you embark on a program of self-treatment, do seek the advice of your physician or a qualified herbalist. Herbal remedies are safe if chosen and used appropriately. Initially, choose one herb only so that you have a clear understanding and appreciation of its action, unless the herbs are in a professionally blended formula. Solgar offers a vast selection of standardized, single herbal remedies that are ideal to start with. 'Standardized' simply means that the herbal products have been processed to guarantee a known minimum quantity of one or more of the major active ingredients.

## GENERAL GUIDELINES

1  If making herbal teas or other herbal preparations, use glass, wooden, china or enamel utensils and containers as metal can react adversely with herbs.
2  Buy from a reputable company and remember that in herbal medicine, a higher price often indicates a superior product.
3  Follow manufacturer's instructions regarding the recommended dose.
4  If any unusual symptoms appear while taking the herb, stop taking it and talk to a qualified expert.
5  As regarding herbs and pregnancy, my message has always been simple: when pregnant do not take anything that is not essential. Do not use basil, rosemary, sage, parsley or garlic that are recommended in various chapters in this book.
6  If there is an organic alternative, always favour this .

## way 3: exercise

Exercise is viewed in very different lights by Chinese and Western societies. Qigong and T'ai Chi are the main forms in China, and are recognized as invaluable aids to ensuring that the energy system is balanced and strong. It is thought that the Chinese were involved in these forms of exercise even before the birth of acupuncture. Gentle to moderate amounts of exercise are recommended to keep the blood and *qi* (*see page 5*) circulating. Not taking any exercise at all can lead to sluggishness and stagnation, which the Chinese see as encouraging the onset of many illnesses. Strenuous exercise is not endorsed, especially at certain times of the year as it is considered to deplete the body and kidney *qi*. For example, when the body energy is at its lowest point during the Winter season, gentle forms of exercise such as walking and swimming are enough to stimulate and encourage the circulatory system to be free-flowing and, at the same time, not drain our vital inner reserves. *(For more on this, see the chapters on organs connected to Winter: the Bladder and Kidneys, pages 127 and 145.)*

In the chapters on specific organs of the body, stretches are included that will help to improve the flow of *qi* along the relevant meridians, so enhancing organ function. Suppleness in the muscles, like in a new sapling, is a sign of a healthy liver (*see page 187*), whereas stiffness and difficulty stretching can indicate that there is stagnation and an imbalance within the organ.

## way 4: reflexology (massage and reflex points)

### WHAT IS REFLEXOLOGY?

Reflexology, or reflex zone therapy as it is sometimes called, works on the principle that all the organs and systems of the body are reflected on the soles and the backs of the feet. The body is divided into 10 zones (corresponding to the 10 fingers and toes) which run up the entire length of the body, five on each side. The right side of the body corresponds with the right foot, the left side of the body with the left foot. 'Twin' organs such as the lungs and kidneys have reflex points on each foot; the colon starts on the right foot and, just as the transverse colon travels horizontally across the body, so the reflex travels across from the right foot to the left foot. When specific reflex points are stimulated, these reflexes increase circulation in different parts of the body, healing, nourishing and energizing the corresponding organs.

The origin of a pressure-point system in the feet can be found some 3,000 years ago in China; the system then spread to India and Tibet. Native tribes in North America also understood the relationship between reflex points and the internal organs, and so practised this therapy based on their knowledge. In China this was superseded by acupressure and acupuncture. Reflexology arrived in Europe in the early part of the 20th century and was developed by Dr William Fitzgerald, who noticed that by applying pressure to certain parts of the body, an analgesic effect could be produced on a corresponding area. Together with Dr Edward Bowers, he produced a book in 1916 called *Zone Therapy* – and so founded the subject as we know it today. Eunice Ingham developed the theory further by concentrating more on the feet, calling this the 'Ingham method of compression massage'. Today she is known as the founder of foot reflexology.

**HOW IT WORKS**

There are many explanations suggesting how reflexology actually works. Certain theories connect it to the nervous system, as there are about 72,000 nerve endings in the feet. It is thought that 'crystals', or waste products that the body has not effectively eliminated, are deposited in the feet. Massaging the appropriate reflex points can help to disperse and dissolve these crystals. These are then removed by the lymphatic system and eliminated from the body. It is also thought that reflexology can help to clear energy blockages in the meridians, the pathways of energy which spread throughout the body like an intricate web (these are discussed further under the Acupressure section overleaf). A rather fun product from Origins is a pair of reflexology socks which have a basic map of the feet on their soles. When you first start to massage your feet these could assist you with remembering the location of the organs.

## TECHNIQUES

The thumb-walking technique is one of the most popular and easiest for the lay person to understand. All you need to do is press your thumb on the reflexology point, then bend the thumb at the first joint to 'walk' it along the whole reflex area, feeling for any 'crystals' or hard, granular lumps. Small circular movements directly over certain reflexes also help to disperse any of these 'gritty' areas that may have formed in the foot. Talc is one of the best mediums to work with; you can finish by massaging the whole area using a base oil (olive, sunflower, apricot, almond) with a few drops of your chosen essential oils.

In Chinese medicine, the feet are very important in terms of the many acupuncture points that begin on the feet. Therefore, it is highly beneficial after working on specific reflexes in the foot to give the whole foot a massage, paying special attention to the area between the toes and the tips of the toes.

Included in the reflexology section (which is actually called Massage and Reflex points in each of the organ chapters) are a selection of some of the major points used in Applied Kinesiology (AK) or Touch for Health. This system corrects imbalances in the body's energy system, having an impact on many levels. Some of the points are recognized acupressure points, but some are specific to this system and are called neuro-lymphatic points. These help to regulate the flow of energy to the lymphatic system and regular massage of these points can release blockages and general congestion. Some schools also teach that the points can be tapped firmly for approximately a minute.

## GENERAL GUIDELINES

1. Never overstimulate a reflex point. Working on an area for approximately one minute will be sufficient. If you buy reflexology sandals then only wear them for a few minutes a day, otherwise the reflexes can be over-worked.

2. Drink several glasses of water after a treatment to flush the wastes out of your system.

3. It is a good idea to rest after massaging your reflexology points so that the body can efficiently eliminate the toxins.

4. Never use reflexology in the first three months of pregnancy, after a heavy meal, or if you have been drinking alcohol. It is not advisable to use reflexology if you are suffering from deep vein thrombosis, diabetes, epilepsy, scar tissue or wounds, varicose veins or other serious illnesses. Please consult a qualified reflexologist if in doubt.

## way 5: acupressure

### WHAT IS ACUPRESSURE?

The system of acupressure is over 3,000 years old and has always been used in China, along with acupuncture, as a way of keeping the body healthy and strong. The Chinese discovered that when pressing specific points on the body for pain relief, this had a beneficial effect on other parts of the body that were not necessarily connected to the points being treated. These points, known as acupuncture points, are located on specific meridians (energy channels) running through the body. The points are named and numbered according to the specific meridian on which they are located.

## HOW IT WORKS

Acupressure is used for pain relief and as an all-round body balancing therapy that can not only release stress and tension held in the body, but support all the body organs and systems. It is therefore an excellent preventative technique. On a very simple level, tension and 'stagnation' (as the Chinese call it) can accumulate around certain acupoints, and this can cause physical symptoms such as muscle stiffness and fatigue. These are due to poor circulation, the build-up of chemicals such as lactic acid in the muscle fibres, and the disruption of the flow of *qi* around the body. Acupressure relaxes the muscles, so improving blood and oxygen supply locally to affected areas, and encouraging the smooth flow of *qi* once again.

## TECHNIQUES

The Chinese use 'anatomical landmarks' such as the bones, and have a measurement known as a 'cun' to locate the points. In Western terms, 1 cun relates to the width of a finger, so elsewhere in this book I have used the term 'one finger width' to help you to locate the right acupoint. Do not worry too much about being in the exact position as it is very likely you will cover the point with your thumb. If there is congestion, the point very often will feel tender to the touch and that is a good guide as to where you should focus your attention!

When you have found the specific point, pressure is generally applied by using the pad of your thumb, or fingertip if you prefer. Keep your pressure on the points relatively light to start with, especially if you are sensitive or your body is fatigued and weak. The principle of 'no pain, no gain' does not apply here, rather wait until your energy and strength have improved and your body can naturally take more pressure. The point can be held for up to a minute or, alternatively, pressure can be applied intermittently by pressing on the point and then releasing the pressure. Small circular massage movements can also be applied to acupressure points. I also use crystals occasionally directly on an acupressure point as they possess electromagnetic properties that can intensify a treatment. Gently press the pointed end of a quartz crystal to increase stimulation and to energize a point. Other crystals have different properties, for example, rose quartz would be an ideal crystal to use on the heart and *pericardium* point as its energy is softer and it is associated with the emotion of love. As acupressure points are bilateral (on both sides of the body), do remember to treat the related point on the other side of the body.

The length of time that the point is held will vary from individual to individual depending on his or her sensitivity and whether the problem is acute. In general, the principle of 'little and often' can be applied, with specific points being massaged or held for up to a minute at a time. If there is extreme pain or discomfort, acupressure can be carried out every two hours until there is improvement. For chronic conditions, acupressure should be done several times a week and continued over a few months for the best results. Another technique included in each acupressure section is called Meridian Tracing (from AK) which ensures that the meridians flow in their natural direction. Once you are familiar with the meridian (there is a diagram in each chapter), it takes only a few minutes a day to trace all your meridians. Alternatively, if you have specific imbalance linking to an organ or meridian, then this is worth tracing several times a day to help strengthen and energize it.

### GENERAL GUIDELINES

1   Never use acupressure if you have consumed too much alcohol, are on strong drugs, after a heavy meal or over a wound or scar.

2   If you suffer from heart trouble or any other serious illness, consult your GP or a trained practitioner before undertaking acupuncture.

3   Avoid acupressure in the early or very late stages of pregnancy and avoid points such as large intestine 4, spleen 6 and gallbladder 20 and 21 throughout pregnancy.

4   Never overstimulate a point or be too heavy-handed with the

pressure on a point. Holding a point strengthens the energy for symptoms of deficiency; rubbing it can sedate excessive energy.

5 Drink several glasses of water (preferably warm!) after a treatment, to help flush waste out of your system.

6 Rest after massaging your points so that your body can efficiently eliminate toxins.

## way 6: aromatherapy

### WHAT IS AROMATHERAPY?

Aromatherapy is the use of aromatic essential oils from flowers, trees, fruits and herbs which help to heal the body on all levels (mind, body and spirit). It has a very strong impact on the whole person and can be classified as a 'holistic' therapy.

It is certainly not a new therapy, although it has become very popular over the last few decades. In fact, Hippocrates once said that 'the way to health is to have an aromatic bath and scented massage every day'. The Egyptians in 4500 BC used the oils in many ways, and ointments containing frankincense and spikenard have recently been found in the tomb of Tutankhamen. In 2000 BC, the Emperor of China wrote about his discoveries regarding the properties of specific plants. Using herbs and oils for healing purposes (along with acupuncture) represents part of the unbroken Chinese tradition which remains to this day. In this century, a French chemist named Rene-Maurice Gattefosse burned his hand accidentally while working in his laboratory. He plunged his arm into a vat of Lavender oil and his burn not only healed quickly, but there was no infection and no scar. He dedicated the rest of his life to researching the amazing beneficial properties of plants and flowers. He wrote a book on the subject called *Aromatherapie,* thus giving this healing system a name it has kept ever since.

Oils have many properties. They can be calming and sedative, analgesic, detoxifying, antiviral and antibacterial; others are revitalizing and stimulating, and even possess aphrodisiac properties. Certain oils and herbs also have an affinity for different organs in the body. For example, garlic goes to the lungs – if you rub a clove of garlic on the soles of your feet, 15 minutes later your breath will smell of garlic!

❋ Oils can penetrate the skin, and as Gattefossé first discovered, extracellular liquids take the oils into the circulatory and lymphatic systems. The oils tend to be carried into the body through the skin via a massage treatment.

❋ Aromatherapy oils are diluted in a carrier oil such as almond, grapeseed or sunflower, then massaged into the skin. As a general guide, 1 drop of essential oil should be mixed with 5 ml of carrier oil. **Check whether the essential oil is classified as weak, medium or strong; if the essential oil is weak, add 2 drops to 5 ml of oil; if medium, add 1 drop to 10 ml of oil; if strong, add 1 drop to 20–30 ml of oil.**

❋ Aromatherapy oils added to the bath are another wonderful way to enjoy aromatherapy; add a maximum of 8 drops as a rule. Use less if the oil is medium or strong (this information is listed with each oil later in the book).

❋ Smell is another powerful way in which we can absorb essential oils. The oils enter the lungs and can affect our nervous system, hormones, emotions and moods. I often fill a spray bottle with water and add a few refreshing oils to stimulate my grey matter while I am researching and writing.

❋ Steam inhalations are excellent for colds and sinus infections. Add 2 to 3 drops of your chosen essential oil into a bowl of hot water, place your head above the bowl and drape a towel over. Breathe in the vapours, coming up for air when necessary!

✳ Oil burners are also readily available today, but do choose one with an ample sized water dish. Otherwise, the water evaporates so quickly that your mixture burns in the water dish, and this leaves a far from pleasant smell! Approximately 5 drops can be added, depending on the size of the dish. Alternatively, you can get plug in burners such as Tisserands Aromastore which is safe to use overnight.

## GENERAL GUIDELINES

1 Certain oils are toxic in concentrated dosages, so if your knowledge of oils is limited, consult a professional aromatherapist who can advise you on what oils would be suitable and in what dosage.

2 The strength of each oil is classified as strong, medium or weak.

3 If using oils in the bath, add them when you have filled the bath, **do not mix them with the hot water directly from the tap**. Keep the bathroom door closed so that the vapours do not escape. Ensure that you relax in the bath for at least 7 minutes before using any soap or shampoo, to get the maximum benefit from the oil.

4 When using citrus oils, it is advisable to mix them in a carrier oil before adding them to your bath water. If you were to add them neat and the drops did not disperse properly, they could burn your skin.

5 Keep oils away from your eyes as they can sting.

6 Purchase the very best oils that you can afford (preferably organic), and ensure that they are both pure and natural, as synthetic versions are now available which do not have the potency and effectiveness of true, unadulterated essential oils.

7 Do not have an aromatherapy treatment if you have consumed alcohol, are on drugs, or after a heavy meal.

8 Do not have an aromatherapy massage if you have a high fever or an illness such as influenza. If you suffer from any other serious illness, consult your GP or a trained aromatherapist before treatment.

9    Avoid aromatherapy in the early or very late stages of pregnancy and avoid using Marjoram, Fennel, Ginger, Peppermint and Rosemary oils. Aromatherapy is beneficial during other stages of pregnancy, although it is best not to massage the abdomen.

10   If you suffer from epilepsy, avoid Fennel and Rosemary oils, and consult your doctor before you begin any treatment.

11   Strong oils such as Peppermint, Camphor, Black Pepper and Eucalyptus can counteract homoeopathic remedies, so do speak to a qualified homoeopath if you are using both therapies.

12   Drink several glasses of water after an aromatherapy treatment to flush the wastes out of your system. It is also a good idea to rest after a massage so that the body can efficiently eliminate toxins and regenerate body tissues.

## way 7: flower remedies

### WHAT ARE FLOWER REMEDIES?

Flower essences are liquids that have been infused with individual plants and flowers. They have the capacity to restore wellbeing to the body on all levels, the physical, mental, emotional and spiritual. It is believed that flowers possess special healing powers due to their energetic and vibrational qualities and that every type of flower has a totally unique energy system and characteristics.

The traditional way of making a flower essence is to put the petals of the flower in a bowl of water and leave them in the sun for several hours to allow the flowers to 'infuse'. This tincture is diluted and preserved with an alcohol such as brandy. Several drops of the resulting remedy are taken on a daily basis.

Flower essences have been used for thousands of years in many different countries. For example, the Native Americans used to match the energies of specific flowers to particular parts of the body that needed healing. In England, Dr Bach, a one-time successful London doctor who became disillusioned with orthodox medical practice, devoted his life after leaving the medical profession to researching the healing power and energy of plants. He eventually isolated 38 different flowers to help heal specific emotional upsets: the Bach flower remedies were born. At Healing Herbs, a company based in Hereford, the flower essence formulas are made according to Dr Bach's original methods by Julian Barnard, a medical herbalist. These genuine essences are highly respected by practitioners due to their quality.

Phytobiophysics is a revolutionary healing philosophy for the ailments of modern society born out of ancient wisdom. An exciting new range of flower formulas which are totally different from the Bach remedies, were developed by Dame Diana Mossop who spent many years researching and matching the electro-magnetic frequencies of healthy cells to those of plants. Thousands of plants and flowers have been collected worldwide and by combing the frequencies of these essences, a range of 20 Phytobiophysics Flower Formulas (abbreviated as FF in each chapter) in pilule form have been produced. These have the effect of regulating energy levels and re-establishing harmony on a very profound level, thereby encouraging the body to recover from trauma. Our joint energies have inspired the creation and development of an exciting range of 14 new formulas for the meridians which are designed to tune the meridians and restore them to optimum function. The Phytobiophysics meridian formulas are included in the Five Element Body Wisdom Organics Flower Formulas and are specially blended to bring balance and energy to each of the five elements. This range contains a blend of these meridian formulas, including the governing or conception meridian in an organic flower or herbal tincture to encourage a resonance with the physical body and organs.

## HOW THEY WORK

Unlike conventional drug therapies, which work primarily on the physical level, the energetic patterns contained within flower essences work best on the emotional, spiritual and mental levels. Flower remedies work in a similar way to homoeopathic remedies in as much as they are a form of subtle energy. The vibrational energy of the plant is captured in the remedy and, when taken orally, helps bring us into a state of harmony by dissolving blockages on the emotional and mental levels (such as worry, fear, anxiety). Once we are in balance again, the state of disease subsides.

### GENERAL GUIDELINES

1  Flower remedies have no side-effects, are not habit-forming, and can be used safely on both adults and children.
2  For a single remedy, a minimum of 4 drops are taken in water or 3 pilules a day. The same is true of Rescue remedy, the classic composite Bach flower remedy for shock and trauma (called Five Flower Remedy in Healing Herbs range) or the Phytobiophysics FF1 Lotus Star for emergency situations and extreme stress.
3  You can take more than one remedy at a time, although some practitioners advocate that you take no more than four different remedies in a specific mixture. If you decide to take several remedies together, take approximately 2 drops of each in a glass of water, or neat under the tongue.

## way 8: affirmations

Your body responds to your thoughts and feelings, so if your intentions are not constructive and in tune with your body's specific needs, then this can have a negative effect on your health.

Affirmations are short, positive statements which you repeat out aloud or silently to yourself to help in the process of change. They can help us to achieve many things including better health and higher levels of self-esteem and self-worth. In the early stages of working with affirmations, one of the most important things that they can do is to help counterbalance negative, self-defeating messages that play in our head. We all suffer from this inner dialogue, fears and worries about our health, our abilities, relationships, self-worth, etc. These worries can be greatly reduced by controlling the way we think. It is rather like erasing a floppy disc on your computer that has irrelevant and obsolete information and over-writing with a dynamic, inspirational and powerful new programme. If we gradually replace negative statements with an affirmation that is supportive and nourishing, this will help retrain and reprogramme the subconscious mind to think in a more positive and constructive way.

Do not panic if at first you find it difficult, just remember that you will be challenging beliefs which you have most probably been carrying since your early years of life! Put effort and passion into them, as saying affirmations mechanically without having any belief or expectations about them will certainly not carry as much power as those said with feeling.

The affirmations in this book are tailored specifically to the organ systems and to reinforcing the emotions that relate to the various organs. You can have great fun making up affirmations, so do not hesitate to try to formulate your own unique statements. Just keep them positive and easy to say. They can be as simple as **I am healthy** or **I feel wonderful** or **I like myself** (better still, **I love myself!**).

Smiling has been proved to boost the immune system and improve health. The physiological changes in the facial muscles are enough to stimulate endorphins, our 'happy pills' from the pharmacy in our head. So try smiling while you say your affirmations; this will boost your mood even more!

## way 9: visualization and meditation

Meditation is an excellent technique for achieving inner peace. Living in a state of inner peace is a key element to nourishing your soul. Through meditation, you can examine fundamental questions about your potential, master the control of your senses and mind, relieve tension and anxiety.

Putting your mind in a completely relaxed state for even a few minutes a day can help each of us deal with life's never-ending string of hurdles. Having a sense of inner calm is one of the prerequisites to achieving and maintaining outer stability and balance.

There is also much research both to support and prove the power of visualization and meditation in overcoming disease and bringing the body back to a state of equilibrium. Visualizations are a way of using the power of our imagination to build constructive, supportive images which help to replace deep-seated negative conditioning and attract a new level of health and wellbeing. They can be used to enhance any area of your life, but the chapters on individual organs focus on visualizations designed to balance and positively transform specific body systems, to enhance and build your general health.

When you try some of the meditations outlined in this book, do not be concerned if you cannot 'see' images. We are all different and some of us can feel, some of us sense – just use whatever process works best for you.

I have also written and recorded an audio CD of guided musical meditations which include visualizations drawn from the wisdom of the five elements which help us to resolve emotions such as grief, anger, worry, fear and lack of self-love. This empowering CD titled *Seasons of the Soul – meditations to balance the body, emotions and soul* contains visualizations that also help you protect yourself from other people's negativity and encourage you to make positive changes in your life. If you would like a copy of this CD, contact me at my PO Box with a SAE or visit my website – www.jenniferharper.com

# what element are you? – questionnaire

This questionnaire is designed to help you find out whether you have a main element (Earth, Fire, Water, Wood or Metal) that is out of balance and needs support. When answering the questionnaire, be as honest as possible and do not reflect for too long over the question, as the most immediate response is normally the most accurate.

---

**Scoring system**

* If you suffer from these symptoms very frequently,
  or you resonate strongly with the emotional picture,              score 3
* If you suffer from these symptoms and emotions regularly,         score 1
* If you suffer from these symptoms and emotions occasionally,      score 0
* If you only have these problems once in a while, or feel
  indifferent towards the question,                                 score -1
* If you have a strong negative response as you never
  experience these emotions or symptoms,                            score -3

---

## EARTH ELEMENT – STOMACH AND SPLEEN

1  Abdominal distension and bloating  ☐
2  Puffiness, water retention and mucus in the body  ☐
3  Tired, aching, heavy and cold limbs  ☐
4  Great fatigue and lethargy  ☐
5  Flabby, weak flesh, lack of muscle tone and strength
   in lower body  ☐
6  Prolapsed organs in lower body, bladder, intestines, uterus  ☐
7  Loose stools and diarrhoea, abdominal gas and flatulence  ☐
8  Poor digestion and assimilation of food, slow metabolism  ☐
9  Pain under the left side of the rib cage near the spleen
   and stomach  ☐

10  Symptoms are aggravated by cold, damp and humid conditions ☐

11  Easily worried and over-concerned ☐

12  Obsessional and compulsive behaviour disorder ☐

13  Upset by change and tendency to become overwhelmed by detail ☐

14  Eating disorders such as bulimia and anorexia nervosa ☐

15  Craving for sweet foods and ice-cream ☐

16  Worse from eating cold foods, sweets and raw fruit and vegetables ☐

17  Appetite imbalance, either voracious or lack of appetite ☐

18  Hiccups and burping, nausea and vomiting ☐

19  Worse between the hours of 7 and 11 a.m. ☐

20  Acid in the stomach, duodenal or gastric ulcers ☐

TOTAL ☐

## FIRE ELEMENT – HEART AND SMALL INTESTINE

1  Palpitations and panic attacks ☐

2  Heart attacks, angina, hardening of the arteries ☐

3  High or very low blood pressure ☐

4  Poor circulation ☐

5  Fatigue with restlessness and anxiety ☐

6  Insomnia and hot flushes in the night ☐

7  Highly coloured complexion ☐

8  Vivid dreams, restless sleep and nightmares ☐

9  Extreme anxiety, emotional unease and lack of joy ☐

10  Hatred and cruel behaviour ☐

11  Lack of self-love and low self-worth ☐

12  Excessive laughter and giggling at inappropriate times ☐

13  Poor muscle tone and swollen abdomen ☐

14  Pain in the throat, shoulder and neck ☐

15  Tennis elbow and frozen shoulder ☐

| | |
|---|---|
| 16 Symptoms are aggravated by excess heat | ☐ |
| 17 Mental confusion and indecision | ☐ |
| 18 Unable to make decisions | ☐ |
| 19 Worse between the hours of 11 a.m. and 3 p.m. | ☐ |
| 20 Hearing difficulties and deafness | ☐ |

TOTAL ☐

## WATER ELEMENT – BLADDER AND KIDNEYS

| | |
|---|---|
| 1 Poor bladder control, frequent urination | ☐ |
| 2 Cystitis and bladder infections | ☐ |
| 3 Puffiness and water retention around the ankles and feet | ☐ |
| 4 Puffiness and dark bags under the eyes | ☐ |
| 5 Infertility and impotence | ☐ |
| 6 Low libido and lack of sexual fluids | ☐ |
| 7 Constant tiredness, lethargy and frequent yawning | ☐ |
| 8 Pain in the lower back, sciatica and lumbago | ☐ |
| 9 Stiffness or weakness of the knees | ☐ |
| 10 Tightness or soreness in the back of the legs and hips | ☐ |
| 11 Pain in arches, soles and heels of feet | ☐ |
| 12 Thin hair, split ends, lack of shine | ☐ |
| 13 Premature greying of hair, loss of hair | ☐ |
| 14 Symptoms are aggravated by cold and damp conditions | ☐ |
| 15 Fears and phobias; timidity and lack of confidence | ☐ |
| 16 Paranoid and suspicious behaviour | ☐ |
| 17 Constant complaining and moaning | ☐ |
| 18 Craving for salty foods | ☐ |
| 19 Soft or brittle, weak bones | ☐ |
| 20 Learning difficulties, slow development, poor memory recall | ☐ |

TOTAL ☐

introducing the therapies

## WOOD ELEMENT – GALLBLADDER AND LIVER

1  Nauseous headaches and migraines ☐

2  Premenstrual symptoms including mood changes and breast tenderness ☐

3  Irregular and painful periods, inflamed genital organs ☐

4  Weak eyesight, sore, tired, dry eyes and spots in front of eyes (floaters) ☐

5  Weak, ridged and splitting nails ☐

6  Stiffness and rigidity in the muscles, especially in the shoulders and neck ☐

7  Problems with tendons and ligaments, lack of flexibility ☐

8  Dizziness and nausea, vomiting brought on by food avoidance ☐

9  Shouting and a loud voice ☐

10  Pain under the right side of the ribcage near the liver and gallbladder ☐

11  Difficulty digesting fatty foods, allergies and low tolerance to alcohol ☐

12  Bitter or metallic taste in the mouth ☐

13  Symptoms are aggravated by wind and draughts ☐

14  Poor organizational and planning skills ☐

15  Frustration, anger, aggression, irritability and extreme nervous tension ☐

16  Jealousy and resentment, unexpressed anger leading to depression ☐

17  Twitches and spasms in the body and muscles ☐

18  Craving for sour foods such as pickles and lemons ☐

19  Worse between the hours of 11 p.m. and 3 a.m. ☐

20  Clumsy and accident prone ☐

TOTAL ☐

## METAL ELEMENT – LUNGS AND LARGE INTESTINE

1   Breathing difficulties, asthma, emphysema  ☐
2   Shortness of breath and fatigue on exertion  ☐
3   Tightness in the chest and a soft voice  ☐
4   Frequent cold and infections, low immunity  ☐
5   Coughing with or without phlegm, throat infections, laryngitis  ☐
6   Sinusitis, sneezing, rhinitis and other nasal difficulties  ☐
7   Excess mucus or, alternatively, dryness and lack of mucus  ☐
8   Excessive or lack of perspiration  ☐
9   Poor sense of smell  ☐
10  Constipation and diarrhoea  ☐
11  Strong smelly odours from faeces or flatulence  ☐
12  Body odour and bad breath  ☐
13  Pain in the chest or in the lower abdomen  ☐
14  Aggravated by heat and dryness  ☐
15  Dryness of the skin, psoriasis and eczema  ☐
16  Grief, pessimism, melancholy, weeping and depression  ☐
17  Unable to 'let go' of the past, bored and apathetic behaviour  ☐
18  Craving for spicy and pungent foods  ☐
19  Worse between the hours of 3 and 7 a.m.  ☐
20  Poor memory and fuzzy thinking  ☐

TOTAL  ☐

Add your scores up for each element: you should have a higher score for one. You can now turn to the relevant chapter to understand more about the organ(s) and what you can do to help yourself.

Due to the nature of the organs and their interrelationships, we can sometimes have several elements producing symptoms. If a clear picture does not emerge after completing the questionnaire, refer to the chapters on the individual organs and see which element(s) are most applicable to you.

# understanding the earth element

The key to

- ※ Balancing Blood Sugar
- ※ Boosting Energy
- ※ Enhancing Digestion
- ※ Increasing Concentration
- ※ Releasing Worry and Obsession

**Partner Organs:** The spleen is paired with the stomach and assists in the 'transformation and transportation' of food and drink. The action of chewing prepares the food for the transforming and transporting work of the stomach and spleen. If food is not properly transformed by either organ, this can lead to a build-up of excessive dampness (water retention and mucus), and congestion. This saps our vitality and further weakens digestion, giving rise to symptoms such as fullness and bloating, lack of appetite, hiccups, loose stools and flatulence, and contributes towards a sluggish lymphatic system.

**Climate:** The climate for the Earth Element is humidity and dampness, both of which can weaken the functions of the stomach and spleen. If your symptoms are aggravated by either type of climate, this is a diagnostic clue to where your imbalances lie.

**Season:** The Earth phase is associated with Late summer – or Indian Summer, as it is often known. It is a time of balance, transformation and neutrality. Describing it in nature's cycles, the Earth phase is when the flowers from Summer have transformed themselves into fruits. It is a time of ripening, just like the key function of one of the Earth organs, the stomach, 'ripening and rotting'. It encompasses everything about the Earth and exemplifies being steady, grounded and secure, with the fruits of the harvest in abundance.

**Colour:** Yellow is the colour associated with the Earth Element and is reflected in the golden hues that are so prevalent in Late summer. When there is a spleen imbalance, a TCM practitioner with a trained eye will be able to detect a yellow tinge in skin tone. A passion for the colour or, conversely, a strong dislike of yellow, can point to an imbalance in this element.

**Time of day:** 7–9 a.m. (stomach) and 9–11 a.m. (spleen) – good times for the stomach to begin digesting food and for the spleen to finish this 'transformation'.

**Body Tissue:** The spleen controls the condition of our flesh and muscles; a firm, toned body is a good indication of strong spleen energy. On the other hand, poor circulation, obesity, flabby flesh, lack of muscle tone, feelings of fatigue or heaviness in the legs, weak muscles and atrophy of the flesh also connect to the Earth Element. Then the texture of the flesh is not smooth; it has the appearance of a watery version of cellulite. Poor circulation is more common in women; one reason this is thought to be so is that menstruation is dependent on strong spleen energy and a monthly loss of blood puts a strain on this organ as it has to generate more blood to replace this.

**Voice sound:** Speaking with a melodic tone points to the spleen and stomach, as a singing sound relates to these organs.

**Sense Organ:** The mouth is the orifice or opening governed by the Earth Element and has a direct relationship with the spleen. The mouth secretes saliva, which is the fluid secretion of the Earth Element; a deficiency of this will prevent food from being digested properly.

**Reflector:** The lips are thought to reflect the strength of the stomach and spleen. When they are moist and rosy, these organs are healthy and strong; when they are pale and dry, these organs need some attention.

**Symptoms of Imbalance:** Obsessions, over-protective, co-dependent sympathy, insecurity, worry, poor memory, excessive dampness of the body (water retention, excessive mucus), weight gain, congested lymphatic system, prolapse and loose stools, digestive disorders, fatigue, nourishment issues, ungrounded and scattered emotionally.

# your body's own food processor

## what your stomach does for you

Stop and think for a moment what happens to your food after you take a bite, chew and swallow. Wouldn't it be interesting to take the path (initially anyway!) that your food takes as it travels through your digestive tract. Your stomach is your food processor and is in part responsible for how your body processes food and nutrients into energy. Conversely, poor digestion can cause a variety of emotional and physical symptoms, such as nausea, vomiting, ulcers, belching, worrying and insecurity, that gnaw away at your stomach.

### TRADITIONAL WESTERN UNDERSTANDING

Digestion begins in the mouth where saliva starts to break down the starches in the food into simple forms of sugar. The saliva moistens the food and makes it easier to pass down through a tube called the oesophagus which leads into the stomach. The stomach receives information from the hypothalamus and pituitary glands in the head which direct the salivary glands, stomach, pancreas and intestines. Powerful acidic digestive juices are then released by the stomach to help breakdown foods. The food is mixed more efficiently by the contraction and relaxation of the muscles of the stomach wall that helps to mix the food with enzymes, turning it into a liquid called chyme. The partially digested food is then released into a tube called the duodenum which is where the gallbladder and pancreas secrete more juices to continue the process of digestion.

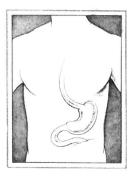

The stomach is a flexible J-shaped sac located on the left-hand side of the body, just beneath the diaphragm. It has the dual function of receiving and digesting foods.

### TRADITIONAL CHINESE INTERPRETATION

| | |
|---|---|
| Element: | Earth |
| Partner organ: | Spleen |
| Climate: | Humidity |
| Season: | Late Summer |
| Colour: | Yellow |
| Time of day: | 7–9 a.m. |
| Body tissue: | Muscles/flesh |
| Voice sound: | Singing |
| Sense organ: | Mouth |
| Reflector: | Lips |
| Taste: | Sweet |
| Emotion: | Sympathy/worry |

## SYMPTOMS OF IMBALANCE

※

### Physical Symptoms

47

Duodenal and gastric ulcers • Chronic gastritis
• Poor or voracious appetite • Nausea, vomiting • Hiccups
• Belching • Colic • Dyspepsia (pain in digestive tract)

※

In TCM the stomach is called the 'Sea of Nourishment' and is the first part of 'receiving and transforming' food and drink into energy. The stomach 'rots and ripens the food', sends the impure to the small intestine and the pure up to the spleen, where the resultant energy is distributed. When this works efficiently, digestion and metabolism are perfect and the appetite strong. This is why some people can get away with eating large quantities of food without gaining weight. Conversely, someone with a weak stomach and digestion can put on 3 kg just by looking at a cream cake!

The stomach energy is downward, so water and nutrients should naturally move downwards, allowing the process of digestion, assimilation and excretion to take place. If the energy is disturbed and moves in an upward direction, symptoms such as belching, hiccups, nausea and vomiting will arise.

※

### Emotional Symptoms

Emotional worries that constantly gnaw away inside
your stomach • Insecurity • Craving sympathy

※

your body's own food processor

※

Food can spend many hours being processed, and emotions can ferment too, creating nausea and tension. A rigid stomach can indicate a resistance to allowing issues to pass through, be digested and finally released. Look at a classic example of how when you are *worried* about an event, your stomach gets tied up in knots and you feel nauseous and sick. If this worry and anxiety is never addressed, but continues to 'gnaw away inside you', the outcome on a physical level could be that the body produces an ulcer.

One simple, cheap and highly effective preventative tool is laughter. Researchers have found that those who laugh frequently are less prone to ulcers and other digestive disturbances. Laughter can stabilize and improve many bodily functions and encourage tissue healing.

There are so many emotive issues that surround food, and advertisers are well aware of this. They use it to its full advantage, seducing us into eating food that titillates our palate but does nothing for our long-term health and vitality. We have a real problem with caring for ourselves and taking the necessary time to feel that we are important enough to nourish ourselves with both enjoyable and nutritional food.

Issues of self-nourishment are often tied up with eating disorders. Food represents mother, lover, affection, security, survival and reward. We often replace our need or desire for any one of these with food as a way of filling the emptiness within. Food is used as a substitute for affection and love, especially during stressful times. Eating excess sweet food (the taste of the Earth Element being sweet) is a way of giving ourselves the sweetness or reward that we may feel nobody else is giving to us. Conversely, starvation regimes express the state of not wanting to nourish or care for ourselves.

The path to breaking some of these addictive patterns is to recognize that there is a problem. The next stage is to make a conscious decision to talk about it to a friend or counsellor, rather than bottling it up. Also, make sure that you then get involved in some form of constructive activity to replace the habit of over-eating or not eating enough. Look at the issues surrounding your lack of self-worth and ways that you can build on this and improve your self-confidence.

# the 9 ways to health

❋ ❋ ❋ ❋ ❋ ❋ ❋ ❋ ❋

## way 1: chinese and natural nutrition

### FOODS FOR THE EARTH ELEMENT

> Grain: millet
>
> Fruit: apricot
>
> Meat: beef (organic)
>
> Vegetable: scallions

The food that we consume is a major contributing factor to the health and wellbeing of the stomach. Equally, our approach to eating food is significant. Traditionally, the Chinese stress the importance of eating meals at regular times, something which is very alien to many people today. Often we eat a meal or snack for the sake of it instead of allowing the body to produce enough hydrochloric acid to digest the food consumed efficiently. Without real hunger, the food that goes into the stomach will not be properly broken down and this will, at some point, create problems.

A simple way of knowing if your body has produced this acid and is ready to digest a meal is to experience and awaken the hungry dragon within who should be bellowing 'feed me'. That hungry feeling before a meal, when you can't wait any longer to be fed, is your body's way of demonstrating that the digestive juices are ready to break down food into

**your body's own food processor**

❋

smaller particles. Very often we eat when the body is not really ready to digest food. We may be stressed or have just had a row and then sit down to a meal. The body cannot digest food efficiently under these circumstances.

Experience has shown that irregular eating habits go on to produce stomach disorders. The following advice is, therefore, as important as the food you eat:

## DIETARY TIPS

1   Do not over-eat, as this prevents the stomach from digesting food properly.
2   Constant nibbling and eating too fast does not give the stomach enough time to digest the food.
3   Eating late at night causes the body to use its *yin* energy (as night is the time for *yin*), putting a strain on the digestive system. It does not like to start the process all over again at night!
4   Under-eating or malnourishment due to strict diets lacking in basic nourishment can weaken the stomach and spleen energy.
5   Eating on the run or while standing up is not advised as it can cause the stagnation of stomach energy.
6   Eating when worried or stressed, no matter how pure and wholesome the food may be, will not do any good and, like eating on the run, can contribute to burning pains, belching and nausea. Eating when angry also has an indirect action via the liver and can cause abdominal distension and pain.

### Foods that strengthen the Stomach and Earth Element
*(also see Recipes, page 207):*

❋   Millet is the grain for the spleen and is one of the oldest cultivated grains known to man. It contains seven of the eight essential amino acids and is said to help improve your physical appearance as well as create emotional balance.

❄ Sweet potatoes, yams and squashes, root vegetables and tubers support the spleen and stomach and are in season in Late Summer, the Earth time in Chinese medicine.

❄ Parsnips are pale yellow and when baked in the oven (and caramelized) have a wonderful sweet taste, the taste associated with the Earth Element. They are high in vitamin A, potassium and calcium.

❄ Sweet potatoes are thought to warm the stomach, strengthen the internal organs and support body energy. They are rich in carbohydrates, beta carotene (which is converted to vitamin A in the liver) and potassium.

❄ Yellow squash is high in all the life-giving minerals and vitamins including vitamin A, calcium, potassium, magnesium and phosphorus.

❄ Other strengthening foods for the Earth Element include apricots, apples (all fruit preferably lightly stewed), chickpeas, cherries, courgettes, cucumbers, dates, grapes, lamb, lettuce, mung beans, oats, peaches, pears, plums, pork, potatoes, raspberries, rice, spinach, strawberries and walnuts.

If you suffer from digestive fermentation and bloating, food combining may be a useful regime to try. This is where you do not eat concentrated starches and concentrated proteins at the same time. There are many books on the market that go into greater detail and also include tasty recipes (*see Suggested Reading, page 304*). For a short cut, another idea is to 'food stack'. This means that you eat the protein part of your meal first so that the concentrated hydrochloric acid juices in the stomach can break the food down more efficiently. Follow this with the starches; so eat the meat or fish followed by carbohydrates such as rice or potato. Remember to chew your food well, as the starches are first broken down in the mouth; this practice alone will help strengthen weak digestion greatly. Keep your intake of sugar, yeast and alcohol low, as this can increase fermentation and bloating. When digestion is poor, eat nuts only in moderation, as they can put a strain on the system, especially if it is weak to begin with, and restrict your intake of fatty foods such as butter and mayonnaise.

**N.B.** A good home remedy if you do suffer from indigestion is to mix a tablespoon of 'live' natural yoghurt containing lactobacillus acidophilus into a glass of water and drink it – this should quickly soothe and remove any irritating pains in the stomach region. Peppermint, chamomile and ginger herbal teas can also help to ease indigestion.

If you suffer from diarrhoea, hiccups and abdominal pains, try eating the following foods:

❋ Star anise, cayenne pepper (in small quantities), fresh ginger, black and white pepper, cloves, chestnuts, ham, garlic, pistachio nut, beef and dates.

❋ Yellow mustard, fennel, nutmeg and cinnamon can be added to the list if there is fatigue, chilliness and a pale complexion.

If you have stomach ulcers:

❋ Avoid spicy foods, alcohol, and herbs such as black pepper, chillies, etc. as they can create too much heat in the stomach.

❋ Cabbage and cabbage juice have long been used to cure stomach and duodenal ulcers – the active ingredient being vitamin U. Fennel, lettuce and potato juice are also helpful.

### Foods that weaken the Stomach and Earth Element:

❋ If you suffer from poor digestion, then try and avoid consuming cold foods and drinks such as ice cream, iced drinks or eat too much raw food. Foods that are classified as having a 'cold' energy in Chinese medicine include soya, tofu, cucumber, melon, bean sprouts, banana, grapefruits and rhubarb. The understanding behind avoiding cold food is that if the food is cold, then the stomach will have to use its own energy to warm to it, and the gastric system has to work harder to metabolize this. Over time this can deplete your vital energy.

## way 2: herbs and spices

※ Meadowsweet is an excellent digestive herb as it can soothe the lining of the digestive tract, reduce symptoms of nausea and excess stomach acidity.

※ Ginger tea is the perfect spice to strengthen digestion and relieve nausea. You can boil dried ginger root for 20 minutes but for a quick fix of ginger, simply grate 2 tablespoons of fresh ginger and fill a mug with boiling water. Put a saucer on top to allow the tea to fully infuse; after 10 minutes strain and drink (although I actually drink the pieces of grated ginger!).

※ If there is heat or inflammation in your stomach, peppermint tea can soothe and help alleviate indigestion.

※ Fennel and dill seeds can also help with indigestion or trapped wind in the digestive tract.

※ Chewing fennel seeds not only supports weak digestion, but has the additional benefit of freshening your breath and preventing tooth decay. Try the Fennel toothpaste by Green People that is 100% natural and organic. It is sweetened by a sweet herb called stevia that is known to inhibit tooth decay and may retard the growth of plaque in the mouth.

※ Cardamom pods work in synergy with fennel seeds and have similar properties to fennel and can help to freshen your breath especially after eating garlic!

※ The herb chamomile is a muscle relaxant that can help to reduce gastrointestinal spasms and can stimulate digestion.

※ Bland herbs such as slippery elm and marshmallow can soothe and calm an irritated stomach. Slippery elm can coat the inside of the stomach, allowing tissue healing and regeneration to take place.

※ Liquorice promotes the healing of the mucous membranes lining the stomach wall. Two derivatives of liquorice root can reduce the size of an ulcer by 70–90% after one month of treatment. High doses should be avoided if suffering from high blood pressure or purchase the deglycyrrhized form.

❋ Body Wisdom Organics produces an Earth Element Organic Herbal Tea Blend that contains chamomile, meadowsweet, dill and ginger.

## way 3: exercise

Some form of movement is essential for the Earth Element, as over-work and excess sitting is thought to weaken the stomach and spleen meridians. However, if there is muscle weakness you probably won't have the stamina for a great deal. Therefore, start gradually by doing 15–20 minutes of gentle exercise every day. Walking in the fresh air and breathing deeply would be a very good start. As your muscles get stronger, you can increase both the duration and intensity of the exercise.

The stretch for the spleen and stomach meridian begins by adopting a kneeling position and placing your hands on the floor. Keeping the spine straight, slowly inhale and put the weight on your hands. Exhale and push your hips towards the ceiling, dropping your head back and trying to relax into the position. Feel the stretch running down the front of your thighs and torso. Remember that it may take many weeks or months to achieve this. Always work at your own pace and ensure that you have warmed the muscles in your body for 10 minutes prior to stretching. If possible, join a local yoga class where you can be guided and personally instructed.

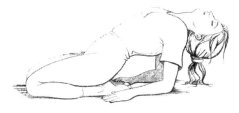

*The Stomach/Spleen Stretch*

## way 4: massage and reflex points

The neuro-lymphatic point for the stomach is found on the left hand side of your rib cage, just beneath your nipple (*see page 56*). Rub firmly for up to a minute.

Massage the reflex points for the stomach, found mostly on the inner side of the left foot. The same area on the right foot can also be massaged. (*See page 23 for massage techniques.*)

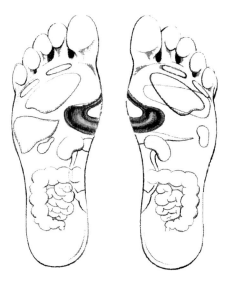

*Reflexology Points for the Stomach (shaded)*

## way 5: acupressure

The stomach meridian begins just below the eye then runs to the jawbone and, after reaching the collarbone, travels inside and so connects with the stomach internally. It resurfaces near the pubic bone and descends down the front of the thigh and along to finish at the base of the nail on the second toe, next to the big toe.

To trace the stomach meridian, take both palms to the starting point of the meridian, just beneath the eye. Run down your face, sweep out along your jaw up to your forehead. Let your hands go down over your eyes to your collar bones, out and down your chest. Follow the meridian line down the body (*see diagram below*) until you reach the end point at your second toes.

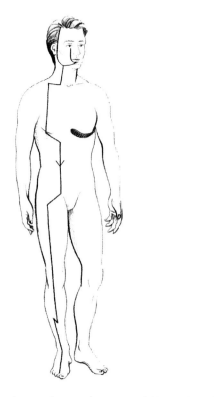

*The Stomach Meridian and Associated Neuro-Lymphatic Point*

The main energizing point on this meridian is located 5 cm beneath the outer part of the knee bone, just on the outside of the shin. This powerful point helps to fight fatigue and support the whole body. It also helps with indigestion and can give relief to other disorders of the stomach, as well as strengthening the whole digestive system. If combined with its partner organ's key point, Spleen 6, the effect will be even stronger (*see diagram, page 76*). When pressing this point, visualize a brilliant golden sunshine colour in and around the point and say the spleen sound, 'WHOOOOOO'.

This is a superb point to burn a moxa stick over (see *'Taking a Deeper Look at Chinese Medicine'* for details on moxibustion), which helps strengthen weak digestion and improve energy levels.

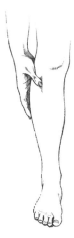

*Stomach 36 Acupressure Point*

## way 6: essential oils

**Caraway:** promotes circulation in the digestive system and has a calming action on the stomach. Helpful for indigestion, pain, belching and bloating. *Strength factor: Strong*

**Cardamom**: for digestive disorders which are caused by nervous strain and worry. Settles feelings of nausea and treats colic, hiccups, indigestion, poor appetite, trapped wind and abdominal bloating. Also a mild brain tonic. *Strength factor: Strong*

**Coriander:** has a warming and drying action which helps to circulate the energy in the stomach and lower digestive tract. Fortifies weak individuals suffering from exhaustion and is useful for nervous depression caused by excessive worry. *Strength factor: Strong*

**Fennel:** Regulates appetite. Fennel tea (as well as the oil being massaged on to the abdomen) has a tonic effect on both the stomach and intestine and can relieve colic, indigestion, nausea, hiccups and trapped gas. *Strength factor: Strong*

**Ginger**: for painful digestion, abdominal distension, loss of appetite, travel sickness (and morning sickness), hangovers and nausea. On an emotional level, it is good for the Earth personality who is over-dependent on others and overwhelmed by self-doubt. *Strength factor: Medium*

**Peppermint:** for acute symptoms such as abdominal pain, indigestion, vomiting, diarrhoea, flatulance and food poisoning. A very weak dilution of peppermint oil can be applied to the stomach area (less than 1 per cent dilution). Drinking peppermint tea helps as well. Also helps with flatulence, food poisoning, travel sickness (keep peppermints in your car for emergencies!). Relaxes and sedates the stomach muscles. Mentally stimulating too. *Strength factor: Strong*

## way 7: flower remedies

**Chicory**: the remedy for 'mothering' types who constantly worry. This love can sometimes turn into possessive and demanding behaviour. Helps to develop the gift of unconditional love.

**White Chestnut**: for times when your mind just will not switch off and your thoughts constantly churn. The remedy can encourage you to get into the habit of assessing problems objectively and talking about your feelings, then deciding on the appropriate course of action to help bring solutions to your problems.

**Dandelion:** FF12 is the key formula for digestive tract disorders and can help with problems such as indigestion, excessive acidity in the stomach, gastritis and is prescribed for the eating disorder bulimia.

**Yellow foxglove**: FF15 is also recommended for someone suffering with eating disorders and helps with digestion and assimilation.

Or try the Stomach Meridian Formula by Phytobiophysics or the Earth Element Flower Formula by Body Wisdom Organics.

## way 8: affirmations

- ❈ My stomach digests food calmly and efficiently.
- ❈ I understand that nourishing my body on all levels is essential and that I am worthy of receiving this nourishment.
- ❈ I trust my stomach to break down the food which I lovingly eat.
- ❈ I am centred and feel satisfied with my life.

*See also the Spleen chapter, page 63, for affirmations that may be used in conjunction with these.*

## way 9: meditation for soul nourishment ...
## nourishing your inner health

Before beginning this meditation, familiarize yourself with the diagrams of the relevant meridians (i.e. for the stomach and spleen).

Imagine yourself lying amongst the fruit trees in an orchard on a warm and mellow day in late summer. The trees are heavily laden with ripened fruit; golden juicy pears, rosy red apples and sweet, succulent plums. As you look at all that nature has to offer at this abundant time of year, feel a sense of appreciation of the rich gifts that this harvest brings. Feel a connection and empathy for the warm earth, supporting and nurturing you.

Now imagine that with every out-breath, a root grows from the base of your spine and smaller roots spread from the end of your toes, going deep into the centre of the earth, securely grounding you. As you inhale, feel your body absorbing energy from Mother Earth. Visualize this energy as a golden liquid and see it filling your entire body, right up to the top of your head. Feel the warmth and energy that this golden colour gives as it is absorbed by your body. This golden yellow resonates with your digestive system and gives strength to the organs like the stomach and spleen that help us to efficiently process food. Food can spend many hours being processed, and so too can emotions which can sit in this area fermenting and brooding, creating nausea and tension. If this worry and anxiety is never addressed and is left to gnaw away inside you, the outcome on a physical level could be that the body produces an ulcer. Go inside and feel whether there is unresolved tension and worry within. Now wrap these emotions in a golden web of light and watch as the golden threads dissolve the anxiety and tension held in the stomach. Feel a great sense of release and peace.

Now focus your attention towards the spleen, found under your ribcage on the left side of the body. When the spleen becomes overburdened we can feel bloated, experience gas, carry excess body weight or water retention and suffer from digestive problems. So imagine this golden liquid travelling through your digestive tract, strengthening and supporting these vital organs. If you suffer from bloating, cellulite, or poor digestion then intensify the golden light in the areas of your body that need extra energy. Feel the light energizing and giving power – clearing blockages and shedding light on any unresolved emotional issues that are connected to nourishment and food.

Be still now and take a moment to reflect on your relationship with food. There are so many emotive issues that surround food, and today more than ever, we are all seduced into eating food that may taste delicious but does nothing for the long term health and vitality of our body. Food represents mother, lover, affection, security, survival, or reward and is used as a substitute for affection and love, especially during stressful times such as relationship separation, loss or bereavement. Food is a way of filling the emptiness within and eating a lot of sweet foods is a way of feeding ourselves the sweetness that we feel no one else is giving us. Try to become more consciously aware of the situations or circumstances that encourage you to use food as a crutch, as awareness is one of the first steps towards healing the past and becoming more integrated. Visualize your body without these problems – see it very clearly radiating health and vitality. Imagine yourself as your ideal you, believe it, feel it and see yourself exuding confidence, joy, energy and health. See yourself being guided to eat more wholesome, nourishing foods that really make you feel vibrant and alive.

Now take your attention to a point just below your left eye that is the start of the stomach meridian. Follow the meridian down as it runs past the chest, travels inside and connects with your stomach before resurfacing near the pubic bone. Charge the meridian with the golden *chi* or energy and feel it flow down the outside of your leg, until it reaches stomach 36, located just below the outer part of the knee. Hold and intensify the *qi* at this point, visualizing the golden light penetrating and energizing this vital point, so increasing the levels of energy in your body. When you feel that you have charged this point enough, allow the energy to move down your leg and finish at your second toe. Now concentrate on the inner side of your big toe just below the nail, where the spleen meridian begins. Send

your body's own food processor

the *qi* along the foot, until you reach spleen 6, a point on the inside of your lower leg, four fingers above your ankle bone. Intensify the *qi* at this point and feel the energy and warmth benefiting your entire body. When you feel that this is stronger, continue up the inside of your leg, then follow up the front of your body to your armpit region and back down to the spleen itself. Now imagine this organ surrounded in golden light. Allow both your stomach and your spleen to absorb this healing light, so enhancing and strengthening their ability to receive and transform Mother Earth's produce into vital energy for you.

Feel waves of golden energy washing over your whole body, filling your mind, body and spirit with a deep sense of satisfaction and fulfilment. Sense your energy becoming stronger and begin to move your fingers and toes, feeling yourself revitalized and grounded ... and in your own time, open your eyes and stretch your body out.

# your body's own energy transformer

## what your spleen does for you

Give credit where credit is due, your spleen regulates many important systems in your body all at once. Behind the scenes your spleen is protecting your body and immune system by regulating several crucial functions including filtering, storing and cleaning blood as well as supporting the lymphatic system. Conversely, in Chinese medicine the spleen is viewed as the main organ responsible for extracting nutrients from food and converting this into energy. According to TCM, physical symptoms of a weak spleen are excess mucus, bloating, poor muscle tone, weak metabolism and low energy levels and the key emotional symptoms are worry and obsession.

### TRADITIONAL WESTERN UNDERSTANDING

The spleen destroys and eliminates any worn-out red blood cells and recycles them into iron for the production of haemoglobin and bile, which is taken to the liver. The spleen stores blood for emergency use; this is what gives the rich purple colour. The spleen is a fundamental part of our lymphatic system and plays an essential role in helping the body fight infections. It produces some of our white blood cells and antibodies that help to neutralize and remove poisonous bacteria and foreign invaders.

The pancreas is located behind the stomach and is connected to the small intestine via a tube. It is part of the endocrine system and is about 15 cm long. It secretes enzymes which help break down the foods in the small intestine and is also involved in balancing blood sugar levels in the body. Pancreatic juice is the only one that digests all three kinds of food: proteins, fats and carbohydrates. The pancreas produces two hormones: insulin and glucagon. Glucagon converts glycogen stored in the liver into glucose (sugar) to raise blood sugar levels and provide an immediate source of energy for the body. Conversely, insulin lowers blood sugar levels by converting excess glucose into glycogen for storage in the liver or into fat to be stored away.

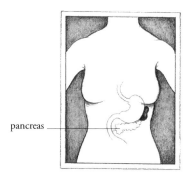

pancreas

The spleen is about half the size of your hand and is composed of soft tissue. It is situated under the left ribcage, just beneath the stomach. It is the largest organ of the lymphatic system.

## TRADITIONAL CHINESE INTERPRETATION

| | |
|---|---|
| Element: | Earth |
| Partner organ: | Stomach |
| Climate: | Humidity |
| Season: | Late Summer |
| Colour: | Yellow |
| Time of day: | 9-11 a.m. |
| Body tissue: | Muscles/flesh |
| Voice sound: | Singing |
| Sense organ: | Mouth |
| Reflector: | Lips |
| Taste: | Sweet |
| Emotion: | Sympathy/worry |

## SYMPTOMS OF IMBALANCE

### Physical Symptoms

Abdominal distension • Bloating and water retention • Prolapse and sagging of the body • Tired body, heavy and aching limbs • Fatigue • Poor co-ordination and dyslexic tendencies • Swollen, cold knees and thighs • Loose stools and diarrhoea • Yellowish face and body • Accumulation of dampness and mucus • Urinary problems and vaginal discharge • Poor memory • Appetite imbalance • Nourishment issues • Aversion to dampness • Poor lymph drainage • Watery cellulite

your body's own energy transformer

In Chinese medicine the pancreas has a very close link with the spleen; the meridian is often referred to as the spleen/pancreas meridian. The spleen's key role in TCM is to transform food, absorb nourishment, extract *qi* and then separate the usable from the unusable parts of food. The transformed food essences create the basis for the formation of body energy or *qi* and blood, which is then combined with the *qi* from the lungs, the two energies mixing to form true energy which is distributed throughout the body.

The state of the spleen is one of the most important factors determining the amount of physical energy a person has; tiredness is a common complaint when this organ is weak. This is because the spleen is the source of life for all other organs. It is in charge of distribution, the transporter of energy. When not functioning efficiently, the body does not receive the energy it needs on the physical, psychological and spiritual levels. The spleen is known as the 'root of post-heaven *qi*', which means it is the major source of all the energy which is produced by the body after birth. As we shall see later, the kidney is the organ responsible for our 'pre-heaven' *qi* or our inherited essence.

The spleen is the organ responsible for transforming food essences into blood and governing the blood circulating throughout the entire body. It ensures that the body is nourished and is said to hold the blood securely in the blood vessels. The spleen energy is also known to have a lifting effect on the body and can hold organs in place, so disharmony in this organ can lead to conditions such as internal prolapse, various types of bleeding (including haemorrhages), chronic diarrhoea and tiredness.

## Emotional Symptoms

Feeling ungrounded and unearthed • Insecurity and
instability • Worry and obsession • Restless sleep •
Needy and selfish behaviour • Confusion and vagueness
• Negative recurring thoughts • Poor concentration •
Scattered feelings • Over-protective of others • 'Stuck'
behaviour

### Helping you understand more about the Mind–Body Link

The emotions corresponding to the Earth Element are sympathy and worry. The phrase 'I need' will be heard often when this element is out of balance. Emotional manifestations of spleen disorders can be seen in the release of negative, disappointed or selfish feelings together with needy and over-dependent behaviour patterns. Individuals who 'vent their spleen' are often trapped in negative recurring thoughts and feelings for both themselves and others. When there is disharmony with the spleen, there can be feelings of loneliness or antagonism towards the rest of the world.

Worrying is an imbalance in the Earth Element and, over time, can develop into obsessional behaviour, mental confusion, dependency and excessive sympathy or pensiveness. This can manifest as the over-protective parent who is constantly worried over his or her children: a 'mother hen' character.

The spleen is said to be the 'residence of thought' or *Yi* and the health of this organ influences our capacity for thinking, studying, concentrating, focusing and memorizing. If the spleen energy is low, this strains the thinking process leading to poor concentration, excessive mental activity, worry and the inability to make decisions.

# the 9 ways to health

✳ ✳ ✳ ✳ ✳ ✳ ✳ ✳ ✳ ✳

## way 1: chinese and natural nutrition

### FOODS FOR THE EARTH ELEMENT

> Grain: millet
>
> Fruit: apricot
>
> Meat: beef (organic)
>
> Vegetable: scallions

The taste for this element is sweet, so if someone has an addiction for sweet foods, or a strong dislike of them, this can be a clue to look at the Earth Element. We in the West tend to have an obsession with sweet food, but the excessive consumption of one type of food to the exclusion of others is not a sensible practice, as a variety of foods is necessary for our health and wellbeing.

The subject of food allergies is a huge topic in itself and is viewed in Chinese medicine as primarily a symptom of poor digestion. It is important, therefore, to build the general health of the body and strengthen the spleen.

Raw food diets are very popular in the Western world, but in the East are not considered to be particularly beneficial. If you are cold or have a weak constitution, a raw food diet can exacerbate this state (*please refer to the interior/exterior causes of disease, page 262*). Some raw food in the diet does provide a rich supply of essential vitamins, minerals and vital enzymes, but long term, if these foods are over-used to the exclusion of other foods, they can deplete the 'digestive fire' (an Oriental term used to describe digestion). Too much cold and raw food will simply make the spleen go soggy and put the fire out, contributing to poor digestion.

It is important to understand that most things are fine in moderation, so if you enjoy juices and fruits, ensure that you also have some warm foods and spices in your diet to create balance. We are all individual and it is important to find out what creates balance and harmony for us personally. Keep an open mind and be prepared to adapt your diet to the seasons, climate and local produce available.

## DIETARY TIPS

1  Reduce your consumption of raw foods and juices in the Autumn and Winter months.

2  Millet is an alkaline, gluten-free grain which does not create mucus in the body. It can, however, be very stodgy if not prepared correctly. It must be soaked overnight and rinsed several times before cooking it for 10 minutes. This prevents it from becoming too sticky.

3  Sweet potatoes, yams and squashes, root vegetables such as parsnips, carrots and turnips support the spleen and are in season in Late Summer (Earth time).

4  Food recommendations to help drain dampness include aduki beans, alfalfa, barley, black pepper, cayenne pepper, celery, chicken, corn, dill seed, fennel, garlic, horseradish, kidney, kidney beans, lemon, lobster, mackerel, marjoram, mushrooms, mustard, mustard leaf, nutmeg, onion, parsley, pistachios, pumpkin, sardines and walnuts.

5  Other foods to strengthen the Earth Element include apples, apricots, cherries, dates, grapes, peaches, pears, plums, raspberries, strawberries (all fruit preferably lightly stewed), chestnuts, chickpeas, courgettes, cucumbers, lamb, lettuce, mung beans, oats, peas, pork, potatoes, rice, spinach and string beans.

6  Black dates can help to replenish *qi* and relieve fatigue.

7  If there is a lot of water in the body, aduki beans, alfalfa, broad beans, celery, clams, fenugreek, lettuce, parsley and seaweed are the best foods to include in your diet.

8   Along with a good natural diet, certain foods can help to cleanse your lymphatic system. These include the herbs nettle and dandelion, leeks and onions from the lily family, fruits such as wild berries, plums, peaches, watermelon and lemons, and vegetables including celery, cabbage and artichoke together with seaweed.

9   If you include foods such as lettuce, it is worth having warm foods with it to help keep the spleen dry, or making a salad dressing with a warming spice such as ginger to pour over the lettuce.

10  Foods which have significant blood sugar-lowering action to support the pancreas are artichokes, Brussels sprouts, buckwheat, cucumber, garlic, green beans, oats, onions, soya beans, legumes, pulses and spirulina or wild blue green algae.

11  Individuals with weak spleens need to ensure that they have adequate amounts of good quality protein in their diet, as this stimulates the metabolism. However, if your digestion is very weak, it is advisable to follow a food combining programme, at least in the early stages.

**Foods that strengthen the Spleen and Earth Element**
*(also see Recipes, page 280):*

As the spleen has an important role to play concerning blood, it is best to ensure that there is a rich supply of good quality 'blood-building' foods in the diet:

❋   The quality of blood can be improved with foods rich in chlorophyll (the green substance found in leafy green vegetables) and algae. For many years I have been aware of the extraordinary nutritional benefits of organic Klamath blue green algae. This supports the spleen as it has a complete nutritional profile that is easily converted into energy. It contains all eight amino acids and is a concentrated source of arginine, an amino acid known to build and support the muscles (which are connected to the spleen). Or try Living Organics Blue Green Energetics Formula produced by Body Wisdom

Organics that not only includes Klamath certified organic Blue-Green Algae (the most nutrient-dense superfood available), but contains herbs such as ginger and cinnamon to assist its absorption, increase energy levels and balance the cool nature of the algae.

Alternatively try the Living Organics Superfood Formula that contains a selection of the best organic 'living' green foods available including the alga, complemented by the addition of such beneficial foods as beetroot, seaweeds, blue-green algae, nettles and ginger. It also includes the four other key herbs and spices that I consider to strengthen specific body systems and balance all of the five elements, together with trace minerals and organisms to promote a healthy colon. All the formulas by Body Wisdom Organics have been developed to synergistically complement each other and can be taken in combination to nourish and support the organs.

- Beetroot is another excellent food for building blood.
- Other foods which strengthen the blood are apricots, kidney and aduki beans, spirulina, red algae (found in silica formulas), nettles, parsley, watercress, eggs, figs and fish such as sardines.
- Flesh foods are well-known blood builders. TCM has it that if a particular organ is weak, you should eat that organ: liver if your liver needs nourishing, kidneys to boost kidney energy, and so forth. If you decide to follow this principle remember that it is essential with offal, and preferable with other meats too, to buy organic.

**Foods that weaken the Spleen and Earth Element:**

- Fatty, refined, artificial foods and sweets. Other foods best avoided or eaten in moderation are raw fruit/vegetables, dairy products and sugar, as they create dampness in the spleen.
- Foods not particularly supportive to the spleen are roasted nuts, wheat, yeast, beer and coffee.
- Avoid excessive consumption of cold liquids and concentrated fruit juices, especially tomato or citrus, as they can weaken the spleen.

# way 2: herbs and spices

※ Ginger is the key spice for the Earth Element as it is a warming stimulating spice and is one of the best herbs to use for digestive disturbances such as nausea, gas, motion sickness and diarrhoea – all symptoms of a weak spleen. A strong cup of Ginger tea (*see page 53*) half an hour before every meal can help to raise your digestive fire allowing your body to efficiently transform food into blood and "*chi.*"

※ Fennel can relieve the pain caused with symptoms such as bloating, flatulence and indigestion. Fennel seeds possess a strong diuretic action and coupled with their ability to help the body to eliminate fats, makes it a helpful weight loss aid. Fennel can help to support our energy levels as it is known to tonify our yang energy and is also useful to help clear excess mucus.

※ Astragalus is known to support the immune system and protect against numerous viruses and has the added advantage of stimulating the metabolism and strengthening digestion.

※ Lycii berries are used in Chinese medicine to build blood and support the spleen.

※ As the spleen likes dryness, foods that are warm and dry are beneficial, as are warming spices such as cinnamon, nutmeg, ginger and cardamom, as well as ginseng, which is said to strengthen the spleen.

※ Liquorice is a spleen *qi* tonic which is often used in formulas in small doses to direct the energy of the formula to the Earth Element.

※ Coriander seeds are excellent for acute indigestion, bloating and gas as they possess anti-spasmodic properties so can ease stomach cramps. The fresh leaves are packed with vitamins and minerals and are more cooling on the body.

※ Look for herbal tincture blends that include Ginger, Coriander, Fennel and Astragalus, such as the Earth Element Organic Herbal Elixir produced by Body Wisdom Organics. In herbal medicine these plants are believed to increase energy levels, aid digestion and nourish the blood. If you are looking for individual supplements, Solgar produces an excellent range of herbs which includes both Astragalus and Ginger.

## way 3: exercise

Proper breathing (*see page 54*), the stretching exercise (*see page 54*) and swimming can have a beneficial effect on the lymphatic system as lymph primarily relies on muscle movement to gently pump it around the body.

## way 4: massage and reflex points

The spleen neuro-lymphatic points are not specific acupressure points but help to stimulate the lymphatic system which is very often sluggish if your spleen is weak. Tapping firmly, or massaging these points for up to a minute can help to strengthen your immune system and boost energy levels. They will often feel very tender (or ticklish!) if there is congestion or you are fighting an infection. Another very powerful point to energize the immune system is the thymus gland which is located approximately 4–5 cm beneath your collar bone on the sternum. Tapping it (and some even recommend thumping it like a gorilla does in the jungle!) for about 30 seconds will help to re-align and stimulate your energy. It is even more powerful when combined with the kidney neuro-lymphatic points (*page 160*).

The reflex points for the spleen/pancreas are situated primarily on the left foot. (*See page 23 for massage techniques.*)

You can also massage the upperside of each foot, starting at the base of your toes and with a gentle but firm pressure, sweep along the foot towards your ankle and repeat five times. This will help to drain and stimulate your lymphatic system. As talc is often the preferred medium for reflexology, why not try a warming talc by Origins called Ginger Dust™ which is talc-free and contains oatflour, cornflour and ginger. Or make your own foot powder using a large teaspoon of powdered ginger to one of cornflour and one of oatmeal. Mix well. If you increase the amount of ginger in this powder, it can help with chilblains if you sprinkle some into your socks.

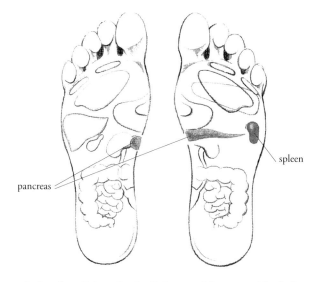

pancreas

spleen

*Reflexology Points for the Spleen and Pancreas (shaded)*

## way 5: acupressure

The ancient Chinese grouped the spleen and pancreas together because they are nourished by the same meridian. The spleen-pancreas meridian is in charge of moving and transforming food, then directing and distributing the resultant energy.

There are 21 spleen meridian points, starting on the outside tip of the big toe nail and running along the medial aspect of the foot, up the inside of the leg, to enter the abdomen and finishing by travelling down to the bottom of your ribs.

To energize this meridian, trace it using your open palm either directly on the skin or up to two inches off your body. Start at the outside of the big toenail and follow the meridian until it finishes at the bottom of your ribcage. You can do both sides at the same time.

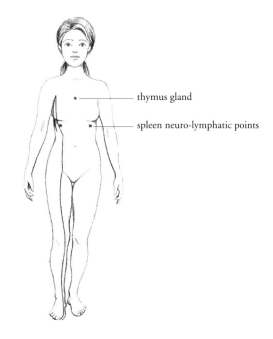

*The Spleen Meridian and Associated Neuro-Lymphatic Points*

**Spleen 6**

This is the most important of all spleen points and is used in spleen deficiency patterns that lead to poor appetite, loose stools and tiredness. However, it can stimulate labour and so *must not be used on pregnant women.*

This point is, more often than not, very tender to the touch and therefore easy to locate. Find the inside of your ankle bone and place three fingers on it; you will find the point above the third finger, just off the edge of the bone. Gently massage the point, or hold it for approximately one minute. Oils will enhance the effect of this treatment.

**your body's own energy transformer**

As it is such a significant point, the benefits are listed below:

- ✳ A major point to dry dampness which can help clear related symptoms such as vaginal discharge and itching, mucus in the stool and cloudy urine.
- ✳ Has a strong influence on blood and can nourish the blood.
- ✳ Excellent for stopping pain, especially abdominal or gynaecological symptoms as it regulates the uterus and menstruation. Heavy, painful periods with clotted blood, or scanty periods will be helped by gently massaging Spleen 6.
- ✳ As Spleen 6 is the crossing point of the spleen, liver and kidney, it can be used to promote smooth flow of liver energy and so is valuable in the treatment of pre-menstrual tension and can support kidney function, so raising vitality and boosting your libido.
- ✳ Also has a strong calming action on the mind and can help where there is indecision, over-thinking or a 'butterfly' mind.

### Spleen 9

This point is located below the knee on the inside of the leg, just below the top of the tibia bone. It is often tender when touched. It is helpful where there is water retention in the legs and abdomen as it eliminates excess dampness in the body; also indicated for diarrhoea or loose stools, vaginal discharge and urinary problems.

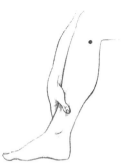

*Spleen 6 (under the thumb) and 9 (just below the knee) Acupressure Points*

Unlike blood which is pumped by the heart, lymph does not have a specific pump to ensure that it travels effortlessly around your body. With the sedentary lives we lead in the twenty first century, congestion is common. Gently massaging your muscles, reflex points, acupressure points and neuro-lymphatic points together with skin brushing, can greatly enhance the performance of your lymphatic system and encourage efficient drainage. Skin brushing is an excellent way to help detoxify the body, as the gentle friction on the skin stimulates the lymphatic system. It is one of the best lymphatic cleansers known, and therefore is supportive to the spleen. When practised daily for a few months it can also improve body tone. This treatment should be carried out on dry skin for about 3 minutes prior to having a shower or bath.

1  Brush the soles as well as the upper sides of the feet using a long-handled natural bristle brush. With long, sweeping strokes, brush up the legs, covering all of the skin's surface area, concentrating on the thighs and buttocks.
2  Put one arm up in the air, allowing gravity to help drain the lymph to the armpit, and sweep down the arm with gentle strokes, drawing the brush towards the armpit.
3  Brush the torso by brushing towards the heart, and when doing the lower abdomen, brush up the right-hand side, just on the inside of the hip bone, across the transverse colon beneath the ribs and down the left-hand side, then gently across the pelvic area to complete the circle. This follows the natural direction of the colon. Repeat.
4  When working near the breast area, brush over the top of the breast, always aiming for the armpit – and remember, be gentle over sensitive areas!

Your skin will become more resilient and you will be able to take more vigorous brushing after a few weeks. Visualize while you do this that your body is being cleansed and purified, with all the toxins being dredged into the lymphatic system to be released in the colon. Stools may contain large amounts of mucus after beginning skin brushing, which is a good sign that the body is beginning to clear away old matter. Skin brushing is subject to 'homeostatic resistance', in other words the body quite simply gets used to it. To override this, it is best to follow a regular daily programme of skin brushing one to two times a day for three months, then reduce this to twice a week – preferably keeping to a regular routine.

The *piece de resistance* is to take a warm shower and follow this with a quick blast of cold water. Apart from being highly stimulating, this encourages the dilation and contraction of the blood vessels and further incites movement of the lymph. You will also feel very invigorated – try it!

## way 6: essential oils

**Bitter orange:** has an affinity with the spleen and stomach and can help to regulate the *qi* where there is stagnation or symptoms such as abdominal discharge and prolapse. *Strength factor: Medium*

**Black pepper:** increases production of new red blood cells. Invaluable for anaemia or after heavy blood loss. *Strength factor: Strong*

**Benzoin:** for lethargy, cold limbs and abdominal bloating. Helps to centre, calm, nourish and comfort those who over-worry. *Strength factor: Weak*

**Caraway:** helpful for bloating and can alleviate dampness by enhancing the spleen's function of 'transformation'. *Strength factor: Strong*

**Fennel:** increases the spleen *qi* and stimulates the lymphatic system. Mild diuretic properties, helping to clear congestion and excess weight. Can help the individual who is prone to over-analysing and has a mind that never goes to sleep! *Strength factor: Strong*

**Frankincense:** good for anyone affected by negative energy or people. Stills the mind, creating peace and calm from within. Has a very strong action on the nervous system and can help to re-build energy levels when they are in danger of weakening the immune system. *Strength factor: Strong*

**Ginger:** has a warming and drying effect on the spleen. Stimulates and tones the digestive system; excellent for abdominal distension, poor appetite, travel sickness (morning sickness too) and nausea. On an emotional level it is good for the Earth personality who can be overwhelmed by self-doubt and is over-dependent on others. *Strength factor: Medium*

**Lemon:** can help to reduce lymphatic congestion, cellulite and obesity. Clears mental sluggishness and strengthens the intellect and mental faculties. Anti-viral properties allow it to support the immune system. A pancreatic stimulant. Can both move the blood and give support to the spleen's function of holding blood and tone in the blood vessels: ideal for haemorrhoids, varicose veins, nose bleeds and even broken capillaries. *Strength factor: Medium*

**Marjoram (sweet):** both relaxes and gives strength in times of weakness and exhaustion. Can pacify emotional cravings and subdue obsessive thoughts and desires. *Strength factor: Strong*

**Myrrh:** for those who are lethargic, cold and are congested both mentally and physically. For indolent wounds that don't heal and for vaginal discharges such as thrush. Excellent anti-fungal, anti-bacterial and anti-inflammatory actions. Centres energies, instilling peace and tranquillity to a worried mind. *Strength factor: Medium*

**Lavender, Bergamot, Tea tree:** stimulate production of white blood cells. *Strength factors: Weak (Lavender), Medium (Bergamot), Strong (Tea tree)*

**Eucalyptus, Rosemary:** also act against a wide variety of bacteria and viruses; increase immune response. *Strength factor: Strong*

For blended oils, Origins Fretnot™ is designed to help you stop fretting and worrying. It contains oils such as orange, lemon and tangerine. If you use this in a bath product, then you could moisturize your skin afterwards with their Ginger Body Oil Spray™. Body Wisdom Organics Earth Element Essential Oil Blend contains ginger, fennel, lemon and marjoram.

## way 7: flower remedies

**Heather:** for individuals who are obsessed with their own troubles, affairs and health issues. Helps them learn to see what lies beyond their personal worries and encourages them to develop greater empathy with others.

**Red Chestnut:** for those who are over-protective towards their loved ones. Helps them to develop the ability to offer guidance and positive support while still remaining partially detached, so allowing them to experience life without projected worries.

**White Chestnut:** for those unwanted thoughts that chase around the mind, leaving you exhausted both physically and mentally and unable to focus on important matters. Sleep patterns are always disturbed, with it being particularly difficult to get to sleep due to the incessant chatter of the mind. Instils tranquillity and peace into the very core of your being.

**Yellow Foxglove:** FF15 is referred to as the sugar balance formula and yellow flowers are thought to help balance the pancreas function and the digestive enzymes.

**Daisy Orange:** FF16 (known to Diana Mossop as the 'Earth' remedy) can help to balance the spleen when combined with Yellow Foxglove FF15.

**Orchid:** FF7 is another formula used to stabilize spleen function.

Alternatively, try the Phytobiophysics Spleen Meridian Formula or the Earth Element Flower Formula by Body Wisdom Organics which contains both the stomach and spleen meridian formulas in a special herbal base.


## way 8: affirmations

These affirmations can be sung if you prefer, as singing strengthens the spleen!

- ❋ My spleen is strong and enables the nourishment of life to reach every part of my body.
- ❋ My spleen glows like the warm yellow sunshine, bathing my body in a rejuvenating and healing light.
- ❋ My thoughts are calm, my mind is focused and I am at peace.
- ❋ My spleen transforms nourishment into golden *qi*, thus increasing my vitality.
- ❋ I am at one with Mother Nature and feel safe and secure.

*See also the Stomach chapter, page 59, for affirmations that may be used in conjunction with these.*


## way 9: meditation for soul nourishment

*See Stomach chapter, pages 60-62.*

# understanding the fire element

The key to

- ❋ Healing your Heart
- ❋ Improving your Circulation
- ❋ Relieving Insomnia
- ❋ Reducing Anxiety
- ❋ Developing Self-love

**Partner Organs:** The organs for the Fire Element are the heart and small intestine. The Fire Element creates warmth, colour and passion in our lives; when we lack fire, we lack emotional warmth.

**Climate:** Heat. Excess heat is injurious to the heart. Someone who adores heat or who on the other hand feels extremely uncomfortable in hot weather, may have a Fire imbalance. Hot and painful joints may indicate that fire has got lodged in an area of the body; fevers and thirst, heartburn and hot flushes indicate this as well. Our body heat is on the surface during the Summer, to try to keep us cool and refreshed. Becoming over-heated and having excess fire is one of the main causes of symptoms of imbalance that can arise at this time of year. To compensate, our diet should consist of cooler, lighter foods during hot weather.

**Season:** Summer, a time when plants have reached their maximum capacity for growth with the hot temperatures and abundant sunshine. We too have more physical energy and often feel the desire to play more sport, do the gardening and go for long walks. It is a time of optimum growth and warmth, like the sun reaching its highest point in the sky. Summer is also an essential time for building and protecting our energy reserves for the remainder of the year. If your energy reserves are low and you feel fatigued, this can mean that the kidney energy is low and that you did not rest enough and recuperate during the Winter. If this is the case, then it is essential that you look after yourself as much as possible in the Summer months, or your energy could be even lower in Winter, leaving you more susceptible to colds and other viral infections.

**Colour:** Red. When there is a heart imbalance, the skin is highly coloured and has a red tone, a passion for the colour red or, conversely, a total aversion to this colour can point to an imbalance in this element.

**Time of day:** 11 a.m.–1 p.m. (heart) and 1–3 p.m. (small intestine).

**Body Tissue:** The heart controls the blood vessels and blood, regulating and maintaining them. The spleen and liver are also involved with the blood, but the heart provides its rhythm and regulation. (The spleen holds the blood, preventing leakages and haemorrhages, and the liver is responsible for the release and storage of blood.)

**Voice sound:** Laughter is the sound for this element: a continuous giggle may be present in the voice, or alternatively there could be a complete absence of laughter and humour. Speech is also ruled by the heart, so incoherence, babbling, stammering and speech impediments, as well as excessive talking, all show that this organ is out of balance.

**Sense Organ:** The tongue. According to ancient texts, the tongue is the mirror of the heart. A TCM practitioner will pay particular attention to the colour of the tongue and to the state of its tip, as this section of the tongue pertains to the heart. Perspiration is the fluid secretion of Fire; the heat is therefore responsible for our sweat. Note how sweating increases during physical exercise when the heart is beating faster to circulate extra blood and oxygen to the muscles. The ancient Chinese believed that sweat could unclog the body, allowing the body/mind to be cleansed throughout.

**Reflector:** By looking at the complexion and observing the texture and quality of the skin, the Chinese could read a lot into the state of the Fire Element. When the complexion is rosy, the heart is strong; when the fact lacks lustre and colour, there may be an imbalance.

**Symptoms of Imbalance:** Common symptoms that can manifest due to an imbalance include issues around love and self-love, nervous exhaustion or excitability, insomnia, hot inflamed joints, redness and disorders involving the heart such as circulation problems, high or low blood pressure, angina and heart attacks.

# your body's own pulse of life

## what your heart does for you

Whereas some organs seem to stay behind the scenes, your heart takes centre stage. While it is often symbolic for love, its state of health and vitality represent the lifeline from which each of us hang on to life. A weak heart can lead to life-threatening physical symptoms such as high blood pressure, hardening of the arteries and heart attack as well as exhibit emotional symptoms that include anxiety, emotional unease and poor self esteem.

### TRADITIONAL WESTERN UNDERSTANDING

The main function of the heart is to pump oxygen-rich blood around the body through the arteries. Deoxygenated blood is sent back through the veins into the heart, where it is sent to the lungs, the carbon dioxide is expelled and replaced with more oxygen. And so the cycle continues. Half the time is spent in activity (systole or contraction of the heart) and half in relaxation (diastole or resting phase). The vitality and health of the heart and circulatory system are fundamental to life and to the integration of all parts of the body. Any weakness present will, quite naturally, have a profound effect on other organs and tissues in the body. Part of the reason for this is because the circulatory system connects to all other body systems and thus has an impact on them all.

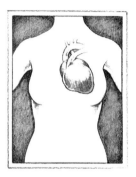

The heart is a muscle roughly the size of your fist. It is located behind the lungs and is protected by the rib cage.

### TRADITIONAL CHINESE INTERPRETATION

| | |
|---|---|
| Element: | Fire |
| Partner organ: | Small intestine |
| Climate: | Heat |
| Season: | Summer |
| Colour: | Red |
| Time of day: | 11 a.m.–1 p.m. |
| Body tissue: | Blood vessels |
| Voice sound: | Laughter |
| Sense organ: | Tongue |
| Reflector: | Complexion |
| Taste: | Bitter |
| Emotion: | Joy/Love |

※

**Physical Symptoms**

※

Hardening of arteries, thrombosis • Heart attacks • Poor
circulation • Low blood pressure • High blood pressure • Hot
and painful joints • Red face or ashen in colour • Angina •
Hot flushes • Weak, irregular pulse • Insomnia • Aversion to
heat • Speech disorders • Poor long term memory

※

In Chinese medicine the heart is part of the Fire Element and is named Emperor of the Body. According to some sources, the heart determines the state and strength of our constitution. Our constitution is primarily related to the kidney energy, but if the heart is strong and the blood in ample supply and able to circulate freely, then the person will be full of vigour and his or her constitution strong. The lungs also play an important supporting role by taking in oxygen and getting rid of carbon dioxide.

According to Chinese medicine, the heart is often seen as the organ most connected with heaven and is described in its spiritual function of 'Housing the *Shen*'. The concept of the *Shen* is a complex one, there being many interpretations. It is probably best translated as 'spirit', although some authorities interpret the heart as the 'residence of the Mind'. A healthy, vibrant person in good spirits would be described as having a good *Shen* or spirit. The *Shen* is often reflected in shining and twinkling eyes.

Next, taking the *Shen* to translate as 'the mind', mental activity is said to reside in the heart, meaning that the heart will affect our mental and emotional health, in particular our memory, thinking and sleep patterns. If the heart is strong, the mind will be both happy and peaceful, memory

※

and thinking will be sharp, sleep sound and we will be balanced on an emotional level. Insomnia, poor memory (in particular long-term memory of past events), forgetfulness, excessive dreaming and incoherent speech problems can arise if the heart energy is weak.

❄

## Emotional Symptoms

Anxiety • Emotional unease • Forgetfulness • Excessive
dreaming • Continuous laughter • Having no joy or
humour • Lack of self love • Poor self-esteem • Cruelty •
Hatred • Over-enthusiasm/agitation • Weak, irregular
pulse • Insomnia • Aversion to heat • Speech disorders •
Poor long term memory

❄

**Helping you understand more about the Mind-Body Link**

Disease is often viewed as a sign that we are becoming more out of harmony with nature. As the heart spends equal time in activity and relaxation, it is important to assess your lifestyle patterns and see if you spend half of your time relaxing and half working. If you don't, it is important to re-evaluate your situation.

Joy is the emotion associated with the heart and the Fire Element. Joy in the positive embodies enthusiasm, fun, happiness and laughter. The Chinese in their wisdom, however, realized that the emotion of joy, either in excess or deficiency, could be just as detrimental to our health as excessive anger. Permanent joy is an impossible thirst and, if sought after through work or play, can put too much stress on the system. In the homoeopathic Materia Medica, excess joy is termed 'mania'. It can agitate the *Shen* or spirit, so triggering insomnia, anxiety, palpitations and other heart problems. Some say that too much joy means a suppression of the other emotions, which all play a part in our make-up – anger, grief, fear

❄

and reflection, and that excess joy at inappropriate moments demonstrates a disharmony of the heart.

Heart troubles can reflect our 'emotional heart', be it lack of self-love, lack of love as a child, difficulties with parents, problems with a loved one in a relationship, etc. Bringing more love into our lives and loving ourselves a little more can go a long way towards helping us to cope with stress.

# the 9 ways to health

## way 1: chinese and natural nutrition

### FOODS FOR THE FIRE ELEMENT

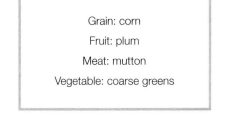

Grain: corn

Fruit: plum

Meat: mutton

Vegetable: coarse greens

The taste corresponding to this element is bitter. The bitter flavour is thought to enter the heart, helping to cool it if it has become overheated as well as cleansing the heart and circulatory system of deposits that have been built up over the years. However, if someone is very weak or deficient, the bitter flavour should be consumed in moderation.

Foods that enhance the Fire function often have colours and qualities that strengthen and stimulate the heart and absorb a lot of sunlight. Such foods include: corn, chives, sunflower seeds, apricots, peaches, plums, red lentils, strawberries and raspberries.

To compensate for hot temperatures in Summer, our diet should be of a cooler, lighter nature. Choosing foods which are easy to digest is important. This is the best time of year to eat salads and fresh fruits which are locally grown and in season. However, those individuals who feel cold on a hot day must try and resist the inclination to eat raw foods, salads and ice cream. If you have a weak immune system, eating these cold, damp foods can encourage the formation of mucus in the Autumn.

**N.B.** It is best to eat foods such as strawberries and other Summer berries only when they are in season.

### DIETARY TIPS

1  Research has indicated that when consumed, refined dietary sugars can be converted into fats and that saturated fats can be manufactured from the presence of starch in your diet. So avoid where possible eating sweet foods such as syrup, confectionery, sugar and refined starchy foods such as white flour, pasta or bread and watch out for their inclusion in a variety of commercial and meat products and ready-made meals.

2  Do not forget that fruit contains sugar in the form of fructose and that wild animals build up their fat reserves for winter by eating available autumn fruits! This is converted into fat to carry the animal through a period where food is scarce. A similar process happens in our own body, although we do not reduce our intake through the winter months! Whereas eating complex carbohydrates such as whole grains provide the best source of slowly released energy, refined sugars do not require the same digestion and are absorbed very rapidly.

3  The metabolism of sugar can promote the creation of cholesterol and saturated fatty acids in the body due to the fact that part of the process in the breakdown of sugar, creates the same building blocks as those needed for cholesterol and fatty acids. The humble oats can greatly help in the fight against cholesterol and a bowl of oat bran

porridge every day can lower cholesterol levels by up to 10%.

4  If you are troubled with poor circulation and suffer with cold hands and feet, remember that warming foods can help to warm the extremities as their action is to direct energy upwards and outwards.

### Foods that strengthen the Heart and Fire Element
*(also see Recipes, page 282)*:

❋ Bitter endive, chicory and dandelion are thought to stimulate the heart and small intestine function.

❋ Asparagus is a supreme Fire food with a bitter taste and has particularly powerful cleansing properties.

❋ Whole grains such as rice and wheat possess bitter qualities in the bran and germ, so it is important to eat them in their natural form, such as brown rice and whole grains.

❋ Longan fruit has the appearance of a reddish raisin and can be purchased from a Chinese Pharmacy. It increases the production of blood and comes highly recommended as a cure for insomnia. It has a sweet flavour and so can be used in sweet congees, desserts and soups.

❋ Fish oils are extremely beneficial to the heart and the whole body as they provide omega 3 fatty acids. You should have at least two portions a week of oily fish such as salmon and mackerel. Another source of omega 3 fatty acids is linseed oil, which is ideal for vegetarians. Virgin cold-pressed vegetable and seed oils provide valuable omega 6 fatty acids which, like the omega 3 fatty acids, are vital for brain function, hormones and general health. (An excellent organic product containing omega 3 & 6 fatty acids in a 2:1 ratio is Udo's Choice oil).

❋ Mung bean tea is another simple yet highly effective way of lowering blood pressure. Pour hot water over 2 tablespoons of washed mung beans and drink first thing in the morning. Keep the mung beans and pour another 240 ml of hot water over them at lunch time and drink. Save the beans yet again, pour another 240 ml of hot water over them and drink in the evening. Mung beans can also be cooked and added to soups or salads.

A deficiency of blood in the body can cause many imbalances, as it nourishes our brain, vital organs, muscles and every part of us. The quality of blood can be improved through diet. (*Refer to page 70.*)

### Calming Foods

As the Shen or spirit is ruled by the heart, it is important to recognize both the foods which settle and support the Shen, and those which weaken it. Sugar, alcohol, tea, coffee, refined foods, large evening meals and food consumed late at night, as well as an excessive amount of ingredients in a meal can all unsettle the Shen. Conversely, lemons have a calming action on the mind, as do whole grains such as rice, oats and wheat. The latter are known for their powerful effect on calming the mind; this is attributed to the fact that these carbohydrate foods raise serotonin levels, an important neurotransmitter in the brain which is known to promote sound sleep and tranquillity. Any food rich in vital minerals, especially calcium, magnesium and silicon, induces a calming action on the spirit and has the additional benefit of giving strength to our bone structure.

Foods rich in calcium include:

※ chlorophyll greens such as watercress, sorrel, rocket, kale, broccoli, parsley, mustard and dandelion greens
※ almonds, sesame seeds (and tahini), brazil nuts, sunflower seeds, pumpkin seeds
※ dried figs, pulses, beans, lentils
※ white fish, canned salmon and sardines (including the bones)
※ olives and oatstraw tea
※ soup made with organic meat or fish bones, with green vegetables and a tablespoon of vinegar added – the addition of vinegar helps to

draw the calcium out of the bones. Eggshells can be added and removed with the bones before serving!

❋ milk is technically high in calcium, but the calcium found in dairy foods comes in an unbalanced relationship with the minerals phosphorous and magnesium, which results in inefficient assimilation and absorption. The nightshade group of vegetables, mentioned earlier, together with citrus fruits can negatively affect calcium balance in the body. Wine, salt and vinegar should be consumed in moderation as these too can bring about a loss of calcium in the body. Fizzy drinks, including carbonated water, lead to excess levels of phosphorus, so disrupting the natural balance of calcium, magnesium and phosphorus, which can result in bone loss.

Foods rich in magnesium include:

❋ green vegetables rich in green chlorophyll (*see calcium list, above, for examples*)
❋ kelp
❋ millet, brown rice
❋ dried apricots and peaches, bananas, dates, avocado, raisins
❋ lentils, peas and beans, cashews and black walnuts.

Foods rich in silicon include:

❋ lettuce, celery, asparagus, dandelion greens, horseradish, spinach, leeks, artichokes, celery, alfalfa, mustard greens
❋ strawberries, apples, carrots, watermelon and cucumber
❋ rice, sunflower seeds, sea vegetables.

Moderation is always the key, so ensure your diet is varied and enjoyable!

**Foods that weaken the Heart and Fire Element:**

❋ As an element, Fire is injured by too much spicy food, animal fat and cholesterol in the blood. Red meat, eggs, dairy food and sugar are all known to raise blood cholesterol levels and prevent an adequate supply of oxygen in the blood reaching the heart. The consumption of these should be greatly reduced or avoided when cholesterol levels are high.

❋ The nightshade family (pepper, aubergines, tobacco, tomatoes and potatoes) are thought to weaken the heart, especially if eaten in a cold, damp climate, like we have here in the UK! They are thought to produce high levels of toxic calcium, which lead to circulation problems such as cold hands and feet. The nightshade group also contains the toxin solanine which may cause symptoms of pain, discomfort and arthritis in susceptible individuals.

❋ If excess alcohol is consumed with these foods, gout, rheumatism and arthritis can develop.

❋ Sudden weight loss regimes and diets must be discouraged as they are particularly harmful to the heart and can put it under great strain. It is common sense to lower the amount of saturated fats in the diet by choosing lean meats and lower fat products and also to cut down on the amount of hidden fats in the diet – as found in cakes, pastries and biscuits.

## way 2: herbs and spices

❋ Cayenne is the key spice for the Fire Element, providing that it is used in small quantities so that it does not over-heat the partner organ to the heart, the small intestine. Cayenne is a superb circulatory stimulant that helps to regulate the flow of blood around the body, as well as strengthen the heart, arteries and capillaries.

- Garlic and onions are helpful in preventing the build-up of cholesterol and garlic has been shown to have a beneficial effect in reducing high blood pressure. The allicin found in raw garlic (the compound that gives garlic its distinctive smell!) has been found to prevent blood platelets from clumping together and forming blood clots, so consuming raw garlic on a daily basis could prove to be helpful in the prevention of strokes and will certainly have a beneficial effect on your blood.

- Olive-leaf extract (Solgar) can help to reduce cholesterol levels and has been shown to lower blood pressure.

- Hawthorn berries have a gentle strengthening action on the heart and their action to lower blood pressure has been clinically proven. It has also been shown that hawthorn berries are effective in the treatment of conditions such as angina and other conditions associated with a weak heart.

- Nettles, one of nature's richest sources of iron, have a diuretic effect on the body and also can have a beneficial effect on both the heart and your circulation. Nettle tea is an easy way to include this valuable herb in your diet throughout the year and the tips of young nettles can be picked in Spring and steamed as a vegetable (like spinach) or added to soups.

- Motherwort is a bitter herb and heart tonic that helps to improve circulation, but should not be used during pregnancy.

- Passion Flower helps to alleviate the symptoms of insomnia without creating a dependency or harmful side effects that sedative drugs can cause. Research suggests that this natural sedative herb can improve both the quality and duration of sleep.

- Chamomile, lavender and oats can encourage a deep and restful sleep, help calm anxiety and help ease states of nervous exhaustion.

- In hot countries, hot spices such as black pepper, red and green chillies and ginger are consumed for a good reason. These are dispersing spices, which open the pores and take heat out of the body, by encouraging sweating. They are ultimately cooling foods in the body, although their taste may at first tell you quite differently!

* Look for herbal tincture elixirs (ideally organic) that include Cayenne, Hawthorn Berries, Motherwort, Passion flower and Chamomile, such as the nutritive Fire Element Organic Herbal Elixir produced by Body Wisdom Organics.

* Body Wisdom Organics produces an organic herbal tea blend for the Fire Element that includes lime flowers, fennel, hibiscus and rose petals. In herbal medicine these plants are believed to clear excess heat from the heart and blood, normalize blood pressure and relieve stress and emotional strain.

## way 3: exercise

Exercise that is of a moderate intensity and adequate enough to get the heart rate up for 30–40 minutes three times a week is recommended to strengthen the heart and cardiovascular system. Deep breathing techniques, visualization, meditation, massage and acupressure are examples of the effective methods available which can help to calm and settle the Shen.

The exercise to stretch the heart and small intestine meridians begins by sitting on the floor with your knees open and the soles of the feet together. Keeping your back straight, inhale and gently lean forward. Exhale as you move into the stretch, seeing if you can lower your knees a little nearer to the floor and bring your head towards your feet. The objective is to try and bring your head, elbows and knees as close as possible to the floor. Remember that it may take many weeks or months to achieve this. Always work at your own pace and ensure that you have warmed the muscles in your body for 10 minutes prior to stretching. If possible, join a local yoga class where you can be guided and personally instructed.

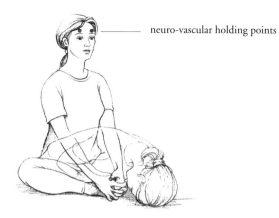

neuro-vascular holding points

*The Heart/Small Intestine Stretch*

## way 4: massage and reflex points

Massaging the sternum close to the heart can help to release tension and tightness around the chest area and ease difficult breathing. Starting at the top of the sternum, work down in small spirals until you reach the tip of the sternum, spending more time on congested, sore areas. The neuro-lymphatic points for the heart on the front of the body can be found in this section that you have been massaging, a few centimetres down from your collar bone on either side of your sternum (*see page 101*). You can also get someone to hold the tip of your sternum and acupressure point Heart 7 for a few minutes. 9–11 a.m. is a particularly potent time to work on issues pertaining to the heart. For particularly sore points or if you feel emotional pain while doing this exercise, make the sound 'HAWWWWWW', which strengthens the heart, and visualize the colour pink or green, whichever you feel intuitively is more suitable.

Using your eyes excessively, as when working at a desk for long hours, can weaken the heart and small intestine meridians, as can emotional stress, which can go on to create more emotional imbalances. One of the best points to help return equilibrium is CV17 (The Sea of Tranquillity).

This is at the centre of your sternum (breastbone) and often feels tender.

To help relieve emotional strain and stress, there are two points located on the bumps on your forehead, 1-2 centimetres above your eyebrows and directly in line with your pupils (*see page 99*). Holding these points, known as neuro-vascular holding points in Applied Kinesiology, while thinking of a person or situation that has caused you anxiety, can help to reduce the level of stress that you are experiencing.

The reflex point for the heart is on the ball of the left foot. Never over-stimulate this reflex, instead gently massage the whole area indicated in the diagram. (*See page 23 for massage techniques.*)

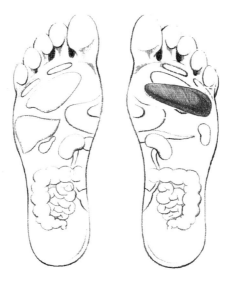

*Reflexology Point for the Heart (shaded)*

## way 5: acupressure

The heart meridian has nine points. It originates at the heart although the first official point (Heart 1) is located under both arms. It runs down the inner arm and finishes on the inside of the nail bed of the little finger nail

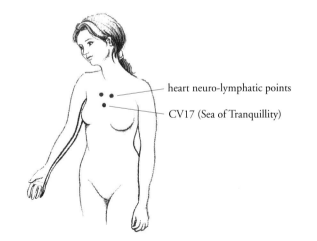

heart neuro-lymphatic points

CV17 (Sea of Tranquillity)

*The Heart Meridian and Associated Neuro-Lymphatic Points*

(Heart 9). It controls the thyroid and influences many menopausal symptoms, such as hot flushes.

To trace your heart meridian, run your palm down the inside of your arm, beginning at the point beneath your armpit. Finish by sweeping off your little finger and repeat on the other side.

### Heart 7

This is the most important point on the heart channel and one of the major acupressure points on the body. Its main action is to calm the mind; it is also used to stimulate poor memory, ease palpitations and anxiety and alleviate insomnia. It is a truly excellent point to calm an over-active, worried mind and to take the heat out of stressful situations.

Heart 7 is located on the inside of the wrist, on the crease. Cupping your wrist, with one hand gently rub the point using your thumb, or alternatively, gently hold the point for approximately one minute. Breathe deeply while you do this, feeling peace and tranquillity flowing into your body and soul.

If you suffer from insomnia then holding the heart points in a warm bath containing Dead Sea salts can be of great benefit as they contain numerous minerals including potassium and magnesium, the latter being known as nature's tranquillizer (*see page 94*). I have certainly found that after a Dead Sea salt bath I sleep very deeply and soundly.

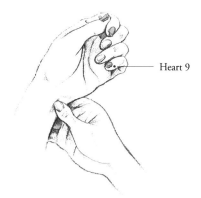

Heart 9

*Heart 7 (on the wrist) and Heart 9 (on the little finger) Acupressure Points*

**Heart 9**

This point can be massaged to calm excess heart heat which has symptoms such as dry mouth, night sweats, insomnia and mental restlessness. Even just massaging the general location of the point on the fingertip by the nail bed is beneficial, as is holding the point between your thumb and finger of your other hand.

It is thought that Heart 7 is more effective on men than women, and that women respond better to a point on the heart protector or peri-cardium channel, Pericardium 7. Pericardium 6 is another major acupuncture point and is one of the best body points to enhance our ability to relate to the outside world, ourselves and our partners. This 'spirit point', as it is known, regulates the energy and protects the heart. It can help to support us in our personal relationships where the heart may have got 'emotionally' injured as a result of difficulties relating to our loved ones.

It is also unrivalled in its action on reducing nausea, vomiting and helping to alleviate travel sickness. To further enhance the effectiveness of this point as an aid to relieve nausea, place a thin sliver of ginger (excellent for nausea) on pericardium 6 and press for up to three minutes.

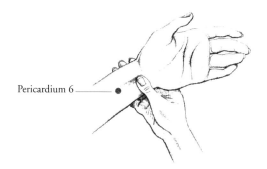

*Pericardium 6 (on the wrist) and 7 (under the thumb) Acupressure Points*

### Pericardium 6

This is located in the middle of the inside of the forearm, approximately two and a half finger-widths away from the wrist crease. Gently hold the point for approximately one minute and feel your anxiety and stress levels diminish.

### Pericardium 7

This point is located on the inside of the wrist, on the mid-point of the crease. Cupping your wrist, with one hand gently rub the point using your thumb, or alternatively, gently hold the point for approximately one minute and feel your anxieties leaving your body. This point is a very powerful aid to comforting and supporting emotions when there are relationship problems. Working on Pericardium 6 and 7 together can enhance the beneficial results.

## way 6: essential oils

**Jasmine:** a beautiful, sensual oil which is very relaxing and emotionally warming. Eases depression and apathy. Helps with relationship problems where sexual difficulties such as frigidity and impotence are involved. Restores confidence and is a good choice for someone with low self-esteem. *Strength factor: Strong*

**Lavender:** has an affinity with the Fire Element, partly due to its ability to clear heat. On an emotional level calms and soothes the Shen in times of stress and exhaustion, so helping with symptoms such as panic attacks, hysteria and insomnia. Invokes peacefulness of spirit and tranquillity of the mind. Can lower blood pressure and ease palpitations. *Strength factor: Weak*

**Neroli:** calms anxiety, nervousness, hysteria and shock; uplifts the Shen. Restores feelings of joy to those who have suffered deep emotional pain. Well indicated for palpitations and high blood pressure; has a cleansing and purifying action on the blood. *Strength factor: Strong*

**Palmarosa:** useful for emotional burnout and nervous tension. Calms palpitations, insomnia and restlessness. *Strength factor: Medium*

**Rose:** one of the most powerful aromatherapy oils for the issues around love; enhances love of the self when we have over-extended ourselves in life. *Strength factor: Strong*

**Rosemary:** promotes circulation, strengthens the heartbeat and raises low blood pressure. Refreshing and stimulating, Rosemary is thought to help with speech impediments (which are connected to the heart and to a Fire imbalance). Can also increase the supply of blood to the brain, and thus has a reputation as an invigorating brain tonic. *Strength factor: Strong*

**Ylang ylang:** a renowned sexual tonic and aphrodisiac often chosen to help with sexual problems such as impotence and frigidity. Helps with palpitations, rapid heart beat, high blood pressure, depression, anxiety, restlessness and lack of joy. *Strength factor: Strong*

**Jasmine** and **Rose Absolute** are known as the King and Queen of essential oils and their price tags certainly reflect this! However, an affordable alternative worth purchasing is Aveda's Singular Notes Line which uses a coconut oil base with the two individual oils.

Origins have spent almost two years working on a range of products designed to help with sleeplessness and include relaxing oils and herbs such as valerian, chamomile, lavender and neroli. The Fire Element Essential Oil Blend by Body Wisdom Organics contains lavender, ylang ylang, chamomile, sweet orange.

## way 7: flower remedies

**Agrimony:** for those who on the surface may appear cheerful but underneath are hiding anxiety and mental torture. Can transform inner pain and suffering by bringing a note of lightness, joy and the ability to laugh at our problems.

**White Chestnut:** for those suffering from insomnia due to unwanted thoughts racing around their head at night. Helps to quiet and calm mental processes, thus allowing the mind to function more efficiently and clearly. Instils an air of tranquillity; can be used to bring about a state of peace and harmony, thus settling the Shen.

**Hawthorn (green):** FF11 is the flower formula for emotional heartache, sadness, blood pressure imbalances and is for those who need a lot of love and support.

**White Rose:** FF2 is the star harmonizer for emotions and when combined with Hawthorn, it amplifies the healing effect, thus speeding up emotional recovery.

**Camellia:** FF3 supports the pericardium or heart protector and can help to stabilize blood pressure.

**Poppy:** FF18 is known as the lifeblood, is a rejuvenating and revitalizing formula that can enhance the circulation and improve the quality of blood, the blood circulation being a vital function which affects the health of our entire body.

**Lotus Vitality:** since *qi* travels through the blood, Flower 1 (FF1) formula amplifies the effect of the formulas.

Alternatively, try the Phytobiophysics Heart Meridian Formula or the Fire Element Flower Formula by Body Wisdom Organics.

You may also find some appropriate remedies for supporting the Fire Element in the chapter on the Small Intestine (*page 121*).

## way 8: affirmations

- ※ My heart joyfully pumps blood to every living cell in my body.
- ※ My heart beats happily with the rhythm of life.
- ※ I fill my heart with peace and joy which I can now share with others.
- ※ I am a loving person who attracts loving relationships.
- ※ I love myself.
- ※ Joy and love fill my body and soul.

*See also the Small Intestine chapter, page 122, for affirmations that may be used in conjunction with these.*

## way 9: meditation for soul nourishment ... opening your heart to love

Before beginning this meditation, familiarize yourself with the diagrams of the relevant meridians (i.e. for the heart and small intestine).

Find a peaceful place to relax and unwind and close your eyes. Focus your attention on your breathing and as you begin to notice it deepening, gently let any thoughts that come into your mind float by like clouds in the sky. For a few minutes, practise the breathing exercise recommended in the Lung chapter.

Imagine yourself lying on a beach on a beautiful Summer's day. The sky is azure blue and the sun radiates warmth and light deep into your body. In the background, you can hear the gentle sound of waves as they roll into the shore. Breathe the warmth and light of the sun and feel it strengthening and nourishing your body. Allow this energy to flow down to your heart and see your heart being supported by a beautiful soft pink colour. Feel the healing that this colour brings to your heart; sense it calming your heart and settling your spirit.

Feel peace and tranquillity flowing through you and easing any heart symptoms you have experienced. Visualize and believe that your heart is getting stronger and healthier every day, and see the pink energy encouraging your blood to flow freely and strengthening your circulation.

The heart is associated with love and joy and your discovery of love will unfold before your eyes if you can look deep inside your own heart to find the love within. Fulfilment lies within and developing self-love will help to bring about positive change in your life as an inner shift always precedes outer change. Only you can take the necessary steps to start loving and forgiving yourself which will lead to the forgiveness of others who have caused you pain. Only then can you begin to remove yourself from the vicious cycle of criticism and rejection. Loving yourself will nourish and heal your soul. By opening your heart to love you will be able to make a stronger connection to your soul and find the love you are searching for to enrich and give meaning to your life. By being a greater source of love and giving love unconditionally to others you will find a greater sense of inner peace and spiritual contentment. Feel your capacity to give unconditional love expand and fill your own heart with love and joy.

Visualize a pink effervescent liquid emerging from your heart and flowing towards your left armpit and travelling along your heart meridian down the inside of your arm until it reaches your little finger. Send energy along this channel and feel the pink effervescent liquid dissolving any congestion in the meridian. Then focus your energy on the outer edge of the little finger nail bed which is the start of the small intestine. Allow the energy to flow up your outer arm and behind the elbow and then see the liquid travelling towards the back of the shoulder. Ensure that you have cleared any congestion before allowing the energy to continue its journey up towards the cheekbone before finishing just in front of your ear. Now, send energy down to your small intestine and allow it to cleanse and purify this area. The warm, pink energy will enhance the small intestine's ability to separate the pure from the impure. This strengthens your ability in life to unleash your true powers of discrimination, so making confused thinking and indecisiveness a thing of the past. Visualize the area in the lower abdomen becoming stronger and believe that your small intestine has the ability to assimilate and absorb necessary nutrients. Feel waves of pink energy washing over your whole body, filling your mind, body and spirit with a deep sense of joy and fulfilment.

If you feel very tired, then intensify the colour and bring in more orange to stimulate the intestine and increase the energy in this vital area of your body. You can focus your energy on a point called the *gate of life* which is a key energizing point on the body situated below your navel. Imagine that the orange liquid is able to support and energize this point, so recharging your physical batteries.

Sense your energy becoming stronger and begin to move your fingers and toes, feeling yourself becoming more alive and awake. Allow your breath now to fill you with energy and passion and in your own time, open your eyes and stretch your body out.

# your body's own sorting house

## what your small intestine does for you

When is the last time you said to a friend, 'By the way, how healthy are your intestines?' Not something we are likely to talk about are we? Most people, however, would be unable to gauge the health of an organ so important to digestion, assimilation and the nutritional quality of our blood. Physical symptoms to watch out for are anaemia, poor muscle tone, pain in the lower abdomen and haemorrhoids.

### TRADITIONAL WESTERN UNDERSTANDING

The small intestine participates in all aspects of digestion, including the absorption, assimilation and transportation of food. It produces enzymes which combine with those sent by the pancreas and gallbladder to help break food down into smaller components. Proteins are thus converted into amino acids, carbohydrates are broken down into simple sugars, and fats into smaller units, allowing efficient absorption to take place.

The inner surface of the small intestine is covered with tiny finger-like projections called villi which increase the area available for absorption. They act like a filter, helping to prevent toxins from being reabsorbed back into the body. Smaller particles of food go through this lining to the liver via the portal vein system, where substances are further processed before reaching the rest of the body. If the small intestine becomes too full of toxins, it can slow the speed and efficiency of the digestive system and impair absorption, as a congested intestine cannot perform all its physiological functions.

One such absorption disorder is coeliac's disease which is caused by an allergy to gluten, the sticky protein found in many grains including wheat. The intestinal lining and villi become damaged and defective, causing serious malabsorption problems and resulting in losses of vitamins and minerals, with diarrhoea compounding the problem. Key symptoms include nausea, smelly stools, abdominal distension, body pain, skin rashes and weight loss.

The quality of our blood – that is, the extent to which it receives adequate nutrition – depends on our diet and the functioning of the small intestine. As the small intestine absorbs iron from our food, which helps to transport oxygen to the cells around the body, it follows that if iron levels are low there will be a corresponding drop in the oxygen-carrying capacity of the blood.

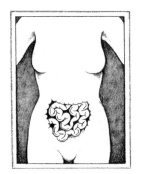

The small intestine is a long, thin tube about 7 metres long; it lies at the base of the stomach and coils through the central and lower area of the abdomen to join with the colon.

## TRADITIONAL CHINESE INTERPRETATION

| | |
|---|---|
| Element: | Fire |
| Partner organ: | Heart |
| Climate: | Heat |
| Season: | Summer |
| Colour: | Red |
| Time of day: | 1–3 p.m. |
| Body tissue: | Blood vessels |
| Voice sound: | Laughter |
| Sense organ: | Tongue |
| Reflector: | Complexion |
| Taste: | Bitter |
| Emotion: | Joy |

## SYMPTOMS OF IMBALANCE

### Physical Symptoms

Poor muscle tone in abdomen • Pain in lower abdomen,
throat or shoulder • Stiff neck and a double chin •
Abscesses in the mouth and upper lip • Tennis elbow •
Frozen shoulder • Difficulty turning head 180 degrees •
Hearing difficulties • Urinary problems • Haemorrhoids
and varicose veins • Coeliac's disease • Anaemia

In Chinese medicine, the two main functions of the small intestine are to 'separate fluids' and to control 'receiving and transforming'. The small intestine receives fluids and food from the stomach after digestion, then

**your body's own sorting house**

'transforms' these by separating the 'pure' from the 'impure': the clean and usable parts of the food from parts no longer needed. The 'impure' parts are sent to the bladder to be released as urine, while the 'clean' parts are sent to the large intestine, not for excretion, but so that vital fluids are reabsorbed into the system. The small intestine has, therefore, a direct and functional relationship with the bladder (which is why bladder problems are included in the 'Symptoms of Imbalance' above).

The small intestine transforms food in coordination with the spleen and the kidneys, although it is important to stress that the small intestine's role is subordinate.

When energy in the small intestine is depleted, you often encounter absorption difficulties and possible malnutrition. Lower back problems can develop, especially around the hara area (located between the pubic bone and navel, and known in Eastern cultures as the source of vitality and health) and there is likely to be fatigue in the hips and legs. Intestinal disorders can also lead to headaches and migraines.

Conversely, too much energy in the small intestine can give rise to stiffness in the neck region in the morning. There is a coldness in the hara due to poor circulation in the lower organs. Cold extremities is another common symptom, as are frequent urination and constipation alternating with diarrhoea.

### Emotional Symptoms

Sadness • Mental confusion • Lack of joy • Critical and cynical • Naive and gullible • Over-thinking • Ambitious but fails to appreciate success • Unable to separate pure from impure

The heart is the partner organ of the small intestine; it is on the psycho-logical level that you can see the closeness of this partnership. The heart governs the whole of our mental life and the small intestine rules our capacity to be clear about our judgements and decision-making.

In Oriental medicine, the small intestine is in charge of digesting emo-tions as well as food, and is known as the Abdominal Brain. The small intestine meridian is a receiving and assimilating vessel involved with nourishment at all levels – emotional, mental and spiritual.

Confusion in our mental state is a common symptom which can arise if the small intestine is unable to sort out the 'pure' from the 'impure'. We will have trouble making clear choices and differentiating between good judgement and poor judgement. This can manifest on a physical level in hearing difficulties (an inability to 'sort out' sounds). The gallbladder is also a decision-maker and, if weak, leads to a lack of courage or conviction to carry decisions through. If the small intestine is weak, however, a decision cannot be made in the first place, as we lose the ability to sort through information or to distinguish between the various options and arrive at a sensible decision. There is possibly no more important role in our lives than to see what is of value and use it to our advantage. What is pure and what is impure, and what are our priorities?

When the small intestine is not in balance an individual becomes ambivalent and is unable to commit to a career, relationship or indeed any course of action that could be sustaining and nourishing. This can ulti-mately lead to self-doubt and frustration as talents are wasted and oppor-tunities lost. Emotions can swing between being overly critical and cynical to, conversely, being naive and gullible. People with a weak small intestine also think too much and control their emotions with their minds; as a result they can experience a deep sense of sadness and lack of joy. If there is excess energy in the small intestine, individuals will be restless, drive themselves hard, overwork, eat fast, find it impossible to relax and will suppress their emotions. They are highly ambitious but often fail to appreciate their accomplishments.

According to ancient Oriental beliefs, negative emotions are expressed in the small intestine by the contraction of particular parts of this organ. Anger contracts the right side of the intestine near the liver; worry affects the upper left side near the spleen; impatience affects the top of the intestine; sadness affects both the lateral sides; fear affects the deeper and lower areas.

# the 9 ways to health

## way 1: chinese and natural nutrition

### FOODS FOR THE FIRE ELEMENT

> Grain: corn
> Fruit: plum
> Meat: mutton
> Vegetable: coarse

### DIETARY TIPS

1   Diet is of extreme importance to the small intestine, which transforms food using a variety of secretions, including enzymes, to break down various components of food into smaller parts to allow for proper absorption. These secretions are mainly produced in the intestine and only remain present when the diet is harmonious and consists of natural foods. If the diet is high in artificial and commercially prepared products then the valuable intestinal flora

population can decline. Acidophilus and bifidus, the beneficial bacteria found in natural 'live' yoghurt and supplements, can be added to the diet to help maintain levels of valuable intestinal flora.

2 If the small intestine is very congested, you should eat boiled white rice for two to three days, ensuring that you chew each mouthful between 50 and 100 times. As already mentioned, 'live' yoghurt and acidophilus powder are helpful too and can heal and soothe the small intestine. Once you have started the detoxification process you will be able to do some gentle massage over the small intestine area.

Refer to the Heart chapter (*page 91*) for more information on foods that support the Fire Element.

### Foods that strengthen the Small Intestine and Fire Element
*(also see Recipes, page 283)*:

* The taste corresponding to this element is bitter, so bitter endive, chicory and dandelion stimulate the functioning of the small intestine.
* Asparagus is a supreme Fire food with particularly powerful cleansing properties, as you can often tell from the strong smell of urea in the urine after eating this vegetable.

### Foods that weaken the Small Intestine and the Fire Element:

* The Fire Element is injured by excess consumption of animal fats and cholesterol in the blood. Too much fat and cholesterol can coat the tiny villi of the small intestine, preventing them from being able to filter nutrients properly. The consequences of this are that the cells in the surrounding area will become undernourished.
* Excessive consumption of hot and spicy foods can ultimately create heat in the small intestine; conversely, too much raw food can contribute towards coldness in the small intestine.

## way 2: herbs and spices

❋ Garlic has been found to help restore the balance of beneficial bacteria in the colon, especially when levels have been depleted due to illness or after a course of antibiotics.

❋ Chamomile and mint herb teas can help clear excess heat from the body and can help to reduce intestinal spasms.

❋ Basil is considered to be unrivalled in its ability to enhance the memory and promote clear concentration.

❋ The culinary herb French Tarragon is also a very good antispasmodic that can help to alleviate intestinal cramps and discomfort.

❋ Coriander and fennel seeds have antispasmodic properties so can relieve abdominal swelling and cramps in your lower digestive tract.

## way 3: exercise

*The specific exercise to stretch the heart and small intestine meridians is described on page 98.*

## way 4: massage and reflex points

The area of a healthy small intestine can be covered with one spread hand and should feel soft and even to the touch. If you press down lightly, it should move gently. If it is full of toxins, there will be a real lack of tone together with an enlargement of the abdomen. Some parts will be slack, others tight, and there will be an uneven quality about the area as it is filled with gas and liquid. This can press downwards and disturb the blood flow in the lower abdomen, resulting in menstrual disorders, varicose veins and haemorrhoids. This excess weight bends the curve of the lower back, pressing on the nerves of the lumbar and sacral plexus, thus inhibiting the messages that the nerves should be getting from the lower abdominal area and organs. This creates muscular tension in the back and legs and can pull at the diaphragm, causing a contraction of the muscles around the ribs. As a result, mucus may be created in the lungs and the lymphatic system may be weakened through lack of movement in the abdomen, thus creating a vicious cycle of toxicity and tension.

Massaging the small intestine helps to eliminate congestion, improves digestion and elimination and allows for the smooth flow of energy.

If the abdomen feels very hard and painful to the touch, work on it only very gently. You may feel knots in the small intestine: these can build up pressure against the nerves that come out of the spine, and contribute to tight muscles. This results in painful contractions of muscles, nerves, lymph and blood vessels. Do not work on these knots directly, but gently massage the whole area first to loosen it, then add a little more pressure directly to the knotty area itself.

Using your eyes excessively as when working at a desk for long hours, or emotional stress, can weaken both the heart and small intestine meridians, which can then go on to create more emotional imbalances. One of the best points to help return balance and equilibrium is CV17 (known as the Sea of Tranquillity – *see page 101*).

Breathing is of the utmost importance to help improve circulation in this area. Place one hand on your navel and the other hand on your chest. Inhale, gently, filling your body like a balloon with air, distending your abdomen like a pregnant woman. If you are breathing correctly, the hand on your abdomen should rise while the one on your chest should remain quite still. Hold the breath for a few moments and then release it, smoothly and calmly, imagining that any tension and toxins are being released with the exhalation.

The neuro-lymphatic reflexes for the small intestine can be found on the inside of the thighs and along the lower curve of your ribcage. Massage the inner thighs and the bottom edge of your rib cage, starting with both hands on the tip of your sternum and with small, circular movements, follow the ribcage around until you reach the side of your ribs.

The reflex point for the small intestine is found on both feet. Reflexologists tend to 'walk' their thumb across this area diagonally or to work from the outer edge of the foot towards the inside in straight lines. *(See page 23 for massage techniques.)*

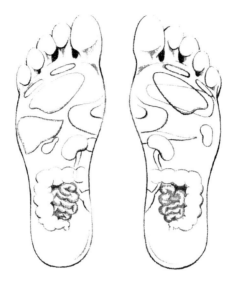

*Reflexology Points for the Small Intestine (shaded)*

## way 5: acupressure

The small intestine meridian starts on the outer edge of the little finger-nail bed, runs up the outer arm behind the elbow, dips over the back of the shoulder to the cheekbone and ends just in front of the ear.

To trace this meridian, run your palm up the outside of your hand, starting at the little finger. Follow up the back of your arm to your shoulder, up and across to your cheekbone and finish by sweeping your palm towards your ear.

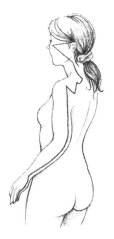

*The Small Intestine Meridian*

### Small Intestine 3

Massaging this point is excellent for relieving a stiff neck, occipital headache, aches down the spine and back. It has a deep effect on the muscles and tendons along the course of the governing vessel and bladder channel, as well as the small intestine channel.

It is located on the outer edge of the hand, approximately one fingerwidth down from the base of the little finger, just beneath the joint. Support your hand at the wrist and, using the thumb of your other hand, massage or hold the point firmly for one minute.

It can clear dampness and also clears the mind, allowing you to make correct and proper choices, as well as giving you the strength to face difficulties in life.

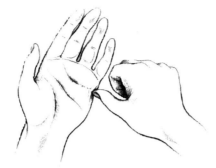

*Small Intestine 3 Acupressure Point*

## way 6: essential oils

**Sweet orange:** an antispasmodic oil that is ideal for digestive disorders and can help to unblock stagnant *qi* when it accumulates in the body. Physically it can also help with symptoms of abdominal distension and pain, flatulence or irritable bowel. Sweet orange is mildly sedative and on an emotional level can help to relax the ambitious workaholic who over-works. Instils an air of buoyancy and joy when inhaled and can be a good oil to help combat insomnia. *Strength factor: Medium*

**Black pepper:** increases local circulation and stimulates a sluggish diges-tive system. Eases pain and spasm. Restores tone to the muscles of the intestines and can aid digestion of heavy food stuffs. *Strength factor: Strong*

**Chamomile:** possesses anti-inflammatory properties and relieves symp-toms of spasm and discomfort in the small intestine, making it an ideal oil for coeliac's disease. *Strength factor: Strong*

**Cypress:** decongests and detoxifies. Due to its astringent properties it helps to constrict and give tone to the veins. *Strength factor: Medium*

**Marjoram:** releases tension knots and tangles in the small intestine. Eases muscular spasm in the lower back. Increases blood flow and promotes circulation, helping to decongest the small intestine while at the same time soothing and relaxing the area. *Strength factor: Strong*

## way 7: flower remedies

**Cerato:** for people who doubt their own judgement and feel they cannot make a valid decision without asking for help from someone else.

**Scleranthus:** for those who just cannot make up their mind and are easily thrown into a state of confusion. Such people are constantly vacillating – even their moods can alternate from happy to sad. Scleranthus fosters clarity of thought and opens us up to our natural wisdom to light and guide our way.

**Vervain:** for those who suffer from excessive small intestine energy leading to a pattern of over-work coupled with a driving ambition which does not allow them to relax or appreciate their accomplishments.

**Wild Oat:** for those who are unable to commit to a career, relationship or any future course of action. Wild Oat is for those with many available opportunities but find themselves unable to decide which path to follow.

**Daffodil:** FF14 on an emotional level is for individuals who are self-critical and are true perfectionists. Physically, it can help with assimilation, detoxification, elimination and purification.

Alternatively, try the Phytobiophysics Small Intestine Meridian Formula or the Fire Element Flower Formula by Body Wisdom Organics.

## way 8: affirmations

❋ My small intestine joyfully absorbs all the nutrients that I need to keep my body healthy.

❋ I am able to assimilate nourishment on every level of my being.

❋ I think clearly, wisely and decisively on all levels.

*See also the Heart chapter, page 106, for affirmations that may be used in conjunction with these.*

## way 9: meditation for soul nourishment ... opening your heart to love

*See Heart chapter, page 107.*

# understanding the water element

The key to

- ❋ Increasing Longevity
- ❋ Dissolving Fear
- ❋ Building Healthy Bones
- ❋ Fulfilling Your Sexuality
- ❋ Boosting the Health of Your Hair

**Partner Organs:** The bladder and kidneys are paired together – theirs is perhaps the most obvious of all coupled relationships. In both Western and ancient Eastern physiological understanding, the kidneys and bladder are connected both structurally and functionally. They make up the water-gate of the body, as the bladder collects urine excreted by the kidneys and holds it until it leaves the body, thus regulating the flow of water.

**Climate:** The Water Element is connected to the North, so it is not surprising that the climate associated with it is cold. Low temperatures and damp conditions can exacerbate and even cause many symptoms pertaining to this element. The kidney energy, like that of the lungs, can be more vulnerable and open to the cold if we have not taken proper care of ourselves over the Summer. People with a weak Water Element generally hate the Winter and really feel the cold. Maintaining your body temperature and wearing appropriate clothing in the Winter months are essential. Make sure you keep your home well heated and be aware that sudden exposure to extreme cold is depleting to the system. Protecting the kidney area is also of vital importance: a scarf worn round your waist will work wonders for your energy over Winter and can protect your kidney 'fire'.

**Season:** Winter. A person with a Water imbalance could experience an aggravation of symptoms in cold weather or may simply detest the Wintertime. Winter is a time for conserving energy, an important part of restoring balance in this vital element, as is proper nourishment, warmth and rest. It is a time of consolidation, of going inwards and hibernating! Psychologically, it is a time of reflection, to contemplate on the year gone by, to assess whether we have met our goals and what lessons we have learned. As symptoms can become more pronounced in Winter, this season can be difficult for some to cope with as the cold can settle deep into the system. Simple advice is to keep warm, rest as much as possible and eat nourishing, warm foods.

**Colour:** Dark blue, although traditionally the colour associated with the kidneys is black, or blue/black. There may be a bluish-black tinge to the skin on the face, especially beneath the eyes, which is the area of the face representing the kidneys, together with puffiness if there is an imbalance in the kidneys. Someone who prefers blue and likes to wear it, or conversely has a strong dislike for the colour, may have an imbalance of the Water Element.

**Time of day:** 3–5 p.m. (bladder); a person with a Water imbalance may find that this corresponds to the time of day when they feel most anxious, tired or irritable. Conversely, if this is your best time of day this too could indicate a slight imbalance, as bladder energy may be in excess. Usually during this time, if there is an urgency to urinate, the body is saying that it wants to let go of the wastes of the day. The time of the kidneys is 5–7 p.m., which may correspond to your lowest energy point in the day with feelings of fatigue and lethargy. If your kidneys are weak, this is a good time of day to rest or meditate.

**Body Tissue:** The kidneys are in charge of the bones and marrow, which means that all bones including the spine, teeth and skull are kept strong and rigid by the energy sent to them by the Water Element. Low kidney energy can result in soft or brittle bones, weak legs and knees and stiffness of the spine, as both bone development and repair depend on the health of the kidneys. The marrow is included as part of the bones, as are the spinal cord and the brain, which is known as the 'sea of marrow'.

**Voice sound:** Moaning. When there is an imbalance in the Water Element, the affected person cannot help but complain, moan and groan about life's little problems; their feelings are clearly detected in their voice.

**Sense Organ:** The ear. Hearing problems are often connected to weak kidney energy.

**Reflector:** The external manifestation of the Water Element is the hair, so a glossy, healthy head of hair shows us that the kidney energy is strong. Conversely, if the hair is dry, broken or split, lacks lustre, goes grey too early or starts thinning or falling out, this reflects weak kidney energy.

**Symptoms of Imbalance:** Key words for the Water Element are fluidity and flow. Any imbalance of our body/mind linked to fluid, such as dryness or thirst, excess or lack of perspiration, urination difficulties, feelings of being overwhelmed or tearful, lymphatic congestion, swelling and bloating, lack of sexual secretions, etc demonstrate that the kidneys are not functioning as they should. The kidneys nourish the brain and influence short term memory in everyday life. When there is a decline in kidney energy as we grow older, the brain does not receive sufficient nourishment. This can lead to memory loss. Learning difficulties also manifest when kidney energy is low. If marrow production is impaired in any way then it can lead to blood deficiency, blurred vision, hearing difficulties and tinnitus. The lower back area is considered by TCM to be the 'Palace of the kidneys', and so a lack of kidney energy may lead to low back pain and pains in the legs.

The bladder is part of the Water Element so the blood and lymphatics also play a significant role as they are all systems that move fluid around the body. Urinary function, perspiration, saliva and tears are all influenced by the Water Element.

# your body's own eliminator

## what your bladder does for you

Are you in touch with your sensitive side? Your bladder wins the award for being the most sensitive organ in your body. It also obviously plays a key role in the elimination of fluid from our body. Symptoms of imbalance to watch out for are poor bladder control, bladder infections as well as complaining, emotional armouring and over-protection. An interesting symptom in TCM is rigidity and stiffness along the back of the body which is where the bladder meridian runs.

### TRADITIONAL WESTERN UNDERSTANDING

The urinary system, which consists of the bladder, the kidneys and the urethra, is one of the body's main methods of elimination. The bladder is in charge of storing and controlling the release of urine, which is excreted from the kidneys. The bladder is able to expand and contract easily due to its elastic muscle fibres, and can hold about 750 ml of liquid. As fluid collects inside the bladder, it builds up pressure until you feel the desire to go to the lavatory.

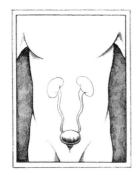

The bladder is a hollow muscular bag located in the lower abdomen and is connected to the kidneys via a pair of tubes called the ureters.

## TRADITIONAL CHINESE INTERPRETATION

| | |
|---|---|
| Element: | Water |
| Partner organ: | Kidneys |
| Climate: | Cold |
| Season: | Winter |
| Colour: | Blue/black |
| Time of day: | 3–5 p.m. |
| Body tissue: | Bones and marrow |
| Voice sound: | Moaning |
| Sense organ: | Ears |
| Reflector: | Head hair |
| Taste: | Salty |
| Emotion: | Fear |

## SYMPTOMS OF IMBALANCE

### Physical Symptoms

Poor bladder control and function • Muscular tension
running up the back • Tightness in back of the legs and
hips • Coolness along the spine and buttocks • Dull,
throbbing headache • Poor circulation • Sciatica or
lumbago • Cystitis and bladder infections • Pale copious
urine or scanty and dark • Lack of perspiration; dryness
and thirst • Stiffness in little toe • Brittleness of joints •
Spasms or pains in calves • Nosebleeds • Headaches at
back or top of head

The bladder can react not only to physical stimuli but also to our emotions. Fear and shock (emotions which affect the Water Element in Chinese medicine) can stimulate the desire to urinate, as can feeling cold, or standing barefoot on cold floors. Bladder infections, as anyone will know who has suffered them, make you aware of the desire to urinate frequently although there is little joy in the amount of urine that is actually passed!

The bladder is an important detoxification and elimination organ; the kidney provides the necessary *qi* to support bladder function. If there is a lack of kidney *qi*, symptoms such as retention of urine or difficulty in urinating can arise. If the bladder is not in balance, any aspect of fluidity within our body/mind may go awry, as Fluidity and Flow are the key words for the Water Element. Symptoms such as brittleness of joints, dryness and thirst, frequency or indeed infrequency of urination, excess or deficiency of perspiration, the lack of flow in thought processes and emotions, and feelings or fears of inundation and being overwhelmed by life

your body's own eliminator

can arise. Adaptability is a key bladder characteristic on many levels, part of the process of flow within the entire mind/body/spirit. If the bladder is not functioning efficiently, the rest of our system will be greatly stressed. In Chinese medicine, excessive sex is said to deplete the kidney energy, and as the bladder is related to the kidneys, this may explain the occurrence of 'honeymoon cystitis'.

## Emotional Symptoms

Armouring, emotional strain • Complaining • Moaning • Highly sensitive • Fears of inundation • Lack of flow in thought processes and emotions • Crying spells • Deep depression • Fear • Feelings of suspicion

### Helping you understand more about the Mind–Body Link

'Armouring' is a key emotion linked to the bladder and this can manifest on many different levels, with the resulting tension corresponding to different layers of muscle. Major surface muscles of the back include the trapezius, latissimus dorsi and the gluteus maximus; important deep muscles include the spinalis and sacro-spinalis. Tension in these muscles is very common and is also associated with great emotional strain.

The bladder, like the kidneys, is affected by fear. A person prone to deep depression and an inability to cope with life situations or change may have an energy imbalance in the bladder. This is particularly true of children, where insecurities and anxiety can lead to bedwetting. In adults, however, bladder disorders are sometimes linked to feelings of suspicion or jealousy over extended periods of time.

# the 9 ways to health

## way 1: chinese and natural nutrition

### FOODS FOR THE WATER ELEMENT

---

Grain: beans and peas

Fruit: dates

Meat: pork

Vegetable: sea vegetables

---

### DIETARY TIPS

1   Eating excess refined carbohydrates will force the body to try and eliminate excess glucose through the urine. Therefore, if you have a urine sample that shows high glucose levels, cutting back on refined carbohydrates may help to normalize this.

2   Too much dampness in the body can cause a variety of problems and can affect major organs such as the spleen, kidneys and lungs. It can also have an impact on the bladder and can contribute to symptoms such as cystitis. Dampness can arise as a result from poor nutrition, eating too much food and excess sweet food in the diet. It is advisable to curtail your consumption of cold, raw foods and excess fluids, roasted peanuts, beer and wheat products. Favour warm foods and drinks and flush the bladder out by drinking boiled water.

### Foods that strengthen the Bladder and Water Element

*(also see Recipes, page 284)*:

- ❋ Kidney beans and aduki beans
- ❋ Barley and buckwheat
- ❋ Sea vegetables are essential to include in the diet and they are easy to assimilate as the protein is almost predigested and, coming from the sea, they have a real affinity with the Water Element. They are extremely high in minerals, and can be added to dishes to increase the nutritional value. Kombu can be put into soups and stews; when you soak beans and pulses adding a piece of kombu to the water and cider vinegar reduces the flatulence that some legumes can bestow! Wakame (tiny strips of seaweed) can be soaked for 10 minutes in water, drained and then added to a stir-fry with rice. If you use a small amount to start with, you really cannot taste it (for those who are repulsed by the thought of eating seaweed!) but will get all those valuable minerals from including it in your diet.
- ❋ Some foods that are known to reduce dampness in the body include green or jasmine tea, onion, turnip, radish, pumpkin, horseradish, Daikon, lemon, mushroom, parsley, alfalfa and mackerel.
- ❋ Fruits of the forest such as blackberries and cranberries are excellent cleansers.
- ❋ Grains such as buckwheat, rice, barley and millet. Millet is alkaline and can help lower acid levels in the body. Buckwheat has warming properties and is known to heat the blood and the whole body. Wheat and rye are the most acidic of all grains and so are best avoided while you are working on raising the alkaline levels in your body.
- ❋ Beetroot is a very cleansing food for the kidneys and bladder and is high in potassium, magnesium and vitamin A.
- ❋ Increase alkaline-rich foods such as fresh fruit and vegetables and millet. Water-rich fruits such as water melons and grapes are said to help prevent kidney stones (although if you suffer from feeling the

cold, consume them only in warmer months); celery, asparagus and kelp all stimulate urination.

*See the chapter on the Kidneys (page 151) for further information on foods to support the Water Element.*

If you have the urge to urinate frequently and there is burning, pain and occasionally blood in the urine, then it is likely that you are suffering from a bladder infection. Cystitis and other bladder infections plague women more often today than any health problem except colds, and are usually caused by bacteria in the urethra and bladder.

Tips to help alleviate cystitis:

- ※ Avoid sugar and sweet foods.
- ※ Drink lots of warm water, as this dilutes the concentration of bacteria in the urine.
- ※ Cranberry juice (approximately 480 ml a day) possesses unique compounds that stop the infectious bacteria from clinging to the cells lining the urinary tract and bladder. Do read labels carefully as some contain high levels of sugar which defeats the object. You can buy an excellent powder from Biocare (UK) which consists of freeze-dried cranberries combined with acidophilus which is highly effective and can also be taken as a preventative measure. You can buy frozen cranberries, but where possible use the fresh fruit. I combine cranberries with carrots, as slow-growing root vegetables are warmer in energy than foods that grow on the surface of the soil such as lettuce. Carrots also help to naturally complement the bitter/sour flavour of the cranberries. (*See the Cranberry and Carrot Soup recipe on page 284.*)
- ※ Avoid caffeine – curtail consumption of chocolate, which contains caffeine and sugar! Tea and cola drinks also contain caffeine.

**your body's own eliminator**

If you have difficulty urinating, try some of the following additional food cures:

❋ Onion and garlic are effective against infections or the urinary tract, as is cider vinegar.

❋ Mash onion and steam it, then apply as a poultice or hot compress to the abdomen below the navel.

❋ Try broccoli and cabbage soup. Soups or broths made with aduki beans, celery, carrots, potato skins and asparagus clear dampness and heat from the bladder area.

❋ Eat peas and spinach.

❋ Kidney beans promote elimination and are excellent diuretics. For swelling due to kidney disorders, make a strong soup with 50 g beans to 1.2 litres of water, cooked down to 240 ml. *Always* ensure that the beans are cooked thoroughly.

❋ Crushed watermelon seeds made into a tea make a useful remedy for the bladder.

## way 2: herbs and spices

❋ The herb uva ursi is very good for cystitis and other urinary tract infections and can be drunk as a tea or taken as a herbal tincture.

❋ Nettles are useful for bladder infections as they can increase the flow of urine so helping to flush excess water and toxins out of your body due to the plant's valuable diuretic properties.

❋ Horsetail is a diuretic herb that is recommended for any inflammatory complaints of the urinary tract such as cystitis. Rich in silica, it also helps to strengthen hair, but high doses should not be used for extended periods of time as it has been suggested that this could irritate the bladder (especially if there is kidney inflammation).

❋ Plantain helps to rid the body of excess uric acid that can accumulate in the kidneys and is a soothing herb that can ease symptoms of a bladder infection.

❈  The above herbs can be purchased individually in a standardized extract form from reputable companies such as Solgar or you can try taking the herb as a fresh juice. The German company Schoenenberger do a whole range of fresh plant juices. Teas such as nettle can be easily obtained from your local health food store and Body Wisdom Organics makes an organic tea blend for the Water Element that includes a selection of the above herbs.

## way 3: exercise

The stretch for the bladder and kidney meridian involves the muscles at the back of the thighs. Sit on the floor and stretch your legs out in front of you. Do not lock your knees but keep them slightly 'soft'. Keeping your lower back straight, gently stretch forwards taking your hands towards your toes. (See *diagram overleaf.*) If you cannot reach your toes, reach to your knees or ankles. Relax into this position and breathe gently and deeply; with each breath, imagine energy moving down your body to the back of your thighs, relaxing the muscles and allowing a deeper stretch. You can try this stretch from a standing position, keeping knees 'soft' and slowly bend forward from the hips letting your head and arms hang. Again, feel the stretch in the back of your legs. Remember that it may take many weeks or months to achieve this. Always work at your own pace and ensure that you have warmed the muscles in your body for 10 minutes prior to stretching. You could also try the spinal rock which is a technique taught at my yoga class which is a wonderful way to release tension held in your spine. Simply sit on the floor, knees near your chest and gently roll your back on to the floor as if you were going to do a backward roll and finish by rocking back into a sitting position. Repeat this several times. If possible, join a local yoga class where you can be guided and personally instructed.

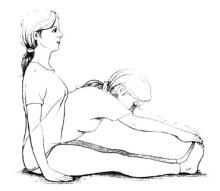

*The Kidney/Bladder Stretch*

## way 4: massage and reflex points

Standing for too long damages the bladder and kidney meridian, which can cause fatigue and low backaches. Traditionally, Bladder 23 is one of the best points to aid tiredness related to the kidney region (*see diagram, page 140*). Make the kidney sound 'WOOOOOO' and visualize a dark blue colour as you rub these points on either side of your spine at around waist height. Another massage technique that not only relieves tension in the back, but also helps to stimulate and flush the lymphatic system is a spinal rub. Ideally, have your partner massage the points on either side of your spine, starting at your neck and work down to the base of your spine. Be gentle around the cervical spine (neck area) but after this you can apply firm pressure and be sure to go in between each vertebrae of the spine, moving the skin to ensure that any congestion is released. Locally pinching the skin can increase blood circulation, so if you find a very tight spot, this technique can help to clear stagnant energy around the individual notches. If you are alone, then have a go at massaging the areas you can reach or try the spinal rock (*page 135*).

The neuro-lymphatic points to support the bladder are located directly on your navel and 1 cm on either side of it. A second set of points on the front of your body can be found running horizontally across your pubic bone.

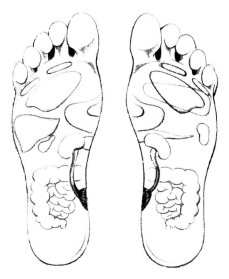

*Reflexology Points for the Bladder (shaded)*

The bladder reflex point is on the inside of both feet near the heel. Trace up the tendon, which is the reflex zone for the urethra until you reach the kidney point. Gently massage this area by 'walking' your thumb from the bladder to the kidney, feeling for any 'crystals'. (*See page 23 for massage techniques.*)

## way 5: acupressure

Acupressure is widely used to improve and maintain kidney and bladder function; used on a regular basis it can be very supportive to these organs. Although the bladder may appear to have a relatively simple task, the points on its meridian relate to every organ and part of the body and have an influence over all the other meridians. The areas covered by this meridian are the neck, shoulders, back, buttocks, back of the thighs and the fleshy part of the calves.

Bladder 1 is located at the inner corner of both eyes; it rises vertically over the forehead and down the back of the neck to the upper back, where it splits into two parallel lines: one 2.5 cm away from the spine and the other 5 cm away. These parallel lines then run down the back, through the kidneys and bladder at the lumbar region of the back, then down the back of the thigh where the two lines join behind the knee. The meridian then continues as one channel along the back of the calf and down the outside of the foot to finish at the outer nailbed of the smallest toe.

It is very therapeutic to stimulate the part of the bladder meridian that runs down the back. This can be done by a partner in a similar fashion to the spinal rub (*page 136*) massaging up and down the channels, noting where the tension knots lie. Alternatively, you could tie two tennis balls into a sock, lie on your back with the balls 2.5–5 cm away from either side of the spine and gently roll the balls up and down vertically over a small section of your back.

You can trace the bladder meridian. Start at bladder 1 and run both hands from this point over the top of your head and neck. Now take your hands behind your back as high as possible up your spine. Run your palms down either side of your spine, buttocks, tracing down over your knees, backs of ankles and sweep off your little toes.

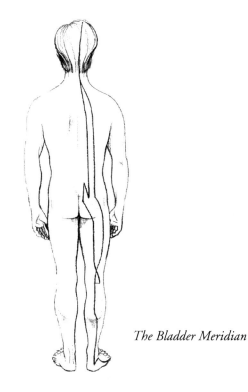

*The Bladder Meridian*

**Bladder 23**

A major point to strengthen the kidney and bladder and boost energy levels. Place your thumbs on either side of your waist and use your middle fingers to find the point, which is on both sides of the spine. Alternatively, rub the back of your clenched fist over this area, gently tapping it to stimulate the region.

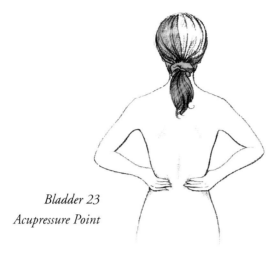

*Bladder 23*
*Acupressure Point*

## way 6: essential oils

**Bergamot:** a powerful disinfectant of the urinary system. Valuable for inflammation and infection. Assists and prevents infections such as urethritis from spreading to the bladder. Must never be used on the skin when in strong sunlight, as it is phototoxic. *Strength factor: Medium*

**Cedarwood:** useful for genito-urinary infections triggered by either cold or damp conditions. A mild diuretic, can also soothe and relieve the pain and discomfort that so often accompanies cystitis. Bestows extra resistance and strength during times of crisis and is a useful 'grounding' oil, helpful as an aid to meditation. *Strength factor: Weak*

**Geranium:** one of the best oils for the tendency towards armouring that is representative of a bladder imbalance. Lets emotional sensitivity in, gently dissolving the barriers we sometimes put up around ourselves and helping us to develop softness and receptivity, while still affording protection to our vulnerable inner self. An anti-inflammatory oil, useful for cystitis, and a diuretic, stimulating the elimination of excess fluid. *Strength factor: Strong*

**Juniper:** one of the strongest diuretic oils available. Purifies and detoxifies. Has anti-infectious properties, ideal for cleansing the body and treating cystitis and urinary tract infections. Prolonged use, however, can over-stimulate the kidneys: use only in moderation and for short periods. Provides emotional strength, support and confidence to those who have isolated themselves due to psychological fears and insecurities. *Strength factor: Medium*

**Sandalwood:** a very powerful urinary antiseptic, yet mild and gentle on the system. Alleviates the discomfort caused by cystitis of a hot and inflammatory nature. Comforting and sedative on an emotional level. *Strength factor: Weak*

**Chamomile**, **Pine**, **Parsley** and **Garlic** oils can also be used to treat urethritis and cystitis; **Tea Tree**, **Myrrh** and **Lavender** help to clear fungal infections which may also be prevalent. The Water Element Organic Essential Oil Blend by Body Wisdom Organics includes Cedarwood, Geranium, Cinnamon and Clove.

## way 7: flower remedies

**Rockwater:** the Bach flower remedy for those who are over-rigid and strict in their approach to life, often becoming so hard on themselves that they do not experience even the simplest pleasures in life and ignore their inner needs, resulting in rigidity in the body and muscles, especially those running up either side of the spine. Can bring out qualities such as softness and the ability to be more adaptable and flexible in life.

**Vine:** for those who are very inflexible and self-opinionated, domineering and possess a will of iron. These traits can lead to extreme stiffness in the body, especially in the back, where the bladder meridian pathway runs. Vine allows such personality types to excel and make the most of their natural leadership qualities, but will help to soften their rigid nature.

**Evening Primrose:** FF13 is the remedy to support the bladder and physical symptoms pertaining to the bladder such as cystitis, frequent urination and bedwetting.

**Daisy Orange:** FF16 combined with FF13 supports the reproductive organs, prostate and bladder.

Alternatively, try the Phytobiophysics Bladder Meridian Formula or the Water Element Flower Formula by Body Wisdom Organics.

You may also find some appropriate flower remedies for supporting the Water Element in the chapter on the Kidneys (*page 163*).

## way 8: affirmations

- My bladder releases all fluid wastes.
- I am adaptable and feel able to open myself to the flow of life.
- I absorb a dark blue healing light, and feel it cleansing and soothing my bladder.
- I am fearless.

See also the Kidneys chapter, *page 165*, for affirmations that may be used in conjunction with these.

## way 9: meditation for the water element ... dissolving fear

Before beginning this meditation, familiarize yourself with the diagrams of the relevant meridians (i.e. for the bladder and kidneys).

Imagine yourself sitting comfortably in a large, old armchair in a room which is lit only by the warm light of a fire. The brilliant embers glow from orange to red and the flickering flames create magical patterns. Outside it is a cold, crisp Winter's evening and bare branches of the trees with a covering of snow are outlined against dark indigo skies. The ground is frozen and hard and all is still and silent. Take your eyes back with relief to the fire and focus on the pictures of mysterious caverns, inviting exploration and leading you into the light. See this as a time of drawing in and consolidating your energy; a time where any dark fears or anxieties can be transmuted into feelings of hope and expectation of the bright future to come with the Spring.

Consciously imagine the deep warmth and glow from the fire and feel this glow now filling your lower back and abdomen. Feel it spreading and flowing around the back of your waist where your kidneys lie. Your kidneys are vital organs in your body which support and give energy to other organs within … so breathe *qi* into them and give thanks to them for providing such support. See them becoming stronger and producing an abundance of vital energy which in turn benefits your entire body. Intensify the warmth and know that it is supporting and regenerating your kidney and life force within. Allow this now to flow down to your knees and feet; feel the deep radiance that this energy brings. Now focus your energy on the base of your foot where the kidney meridian begins. Begin to build and intensify the energy or *qi* at kidney 1 on the sole of your foot. Imagine a deep, dark blue liquid building here and consciously begin to channel this through the kidney meridian taking it around the inner ankle and then see it travel up the inner part of your leg towards your abdomen. As it continues towards your navel, concentrate the *qi* and sense it filling the whole area including your kidneys with healing golden light. Feel the energy expanding and filling the pelvis.

Allow this to restore your very essence and being; to replenish and enhance your sexual *qi* which according to Eastern medicine, is supported by your kidneys. Then allow the dark blue liquid to continue its journey to the end of the meridian by allowing it to flow to a point just beneath your collar bone. Transmute the dark blue liquid into a vibrant golden ball of light and allow this energy to build beneath both your collar bones.

Visualize it cleansing all parts of you and dissolving your fears. As your fears melt away, feel courage and strength building within. Feel empowered! Let this sensation soak into your consciousness and enjoy the positive feelings that being empowered gives you. Now, take this energy to the inner corner of your eye, which is the start of the bladder meridian. Imagine the dark blue liquid once again flowing through the meridian, clearing any blockages as it flows across the top of your head and down the back of your neck. Visualize it then dividing into the two parallel channels that run down either side of your spine. Imagine that the healing blue liquid dissolves any obstruction or rigidity held in your back. Can you feel areas in your spine that feel blocked and tense? Or emotionally can you relate to feeling stiff and inflexible in certain areas of your life? Intensify the energy and allow it to diffuse and clear these blockages, allowing any negativity that has been released to flow down the body and into the earth where it is transmuted. Allow the dark blue liquid to continue flowing down the meridian pathway in the back of your legs, through your knees and into your feet until it reaches the end of the meridian at the little toes. As it reaches this point, take a deep breath and release any final traces of tension that you may be holding in the back of your body ... let the stiffness melt into the blue liquid and allow it to flow into the earth, where it is transmuted. Give thanks for this.

If you wish to sleep now, stay in this deeply relaxed state of being and know that you will wake in the morning feeling refreshed and rejuvenated. If however, you want to wake, then in your own time, sense your energy becoming stronger and begin to move your fingers and toes. Take a deep breath in and feel new life and power enter your body. Open your eyes and stretch your body out feeling yourself rejuvenated and regenerated.

# your body's own sex and energy centre

## what your kidneys do for you

The award for the single most important organ affecting the length and quality of your life goes to ... the kidneys. Even the heart cannot provide such a diverse and crucial list of functions for the body such as filtering blood, elimination and removing poison. The Chinese understanding is very interesting too in that it establishes the kidneys as our sex and energy centre. Physical symptoms to watch out for are premature ageing, impotence and urination problems. Emotional symptoms from traditional Chinese medicine include fear, lack of willpower and depression.

### TRADITIONAL WESTERN UNDERSTANDING

The main function of the kidneys according to Western physiology is to filter blood and body fluids. A large portion of the body's wastes are eliminated through the kidneys, as they help to remove poisons from the liver. High levels of toxins in the body put the kidneys under pressure.

According to Western medicine, severe imbalances in the kidneys can cause cystitis and other bladder disorders and even prostate disorders in men. If the kidneys cannot purify the body when toxic waste levels are too high, calcium and other by-products may be deposited in the kidneys and other vital organs, possibly contributing to arterial sclerosis, cell degeneration and kidney stones. It is also thought that kidney stones can develop when the moisture level in the body is too low; this is one of the reasons why it is recommended that everyone should drink several glasses of pure water every day.

The heart and kidneys have a close relationship, as blood and waste is separated and the purified blood returns to the heart to be circulated around the body. Approximately 5 litres per hour of blood flow through the kidneys, to be broken down into nutritional components. Too much salt in the diet can contribute to high blood pressure, as the kidneys help to adjust blood pressure.

The kidneys are connected to the adrenal glands, which sit on top of each kidney (adrenal being the medical term for kidney-related), and to adrenaline, a hormone released at critical and stressful times. With allergies on the increase, coupled with stress in our daily lives, the kidneys and adrenals are often overworked, giving rise to a wide range of symptoms including fatigue.

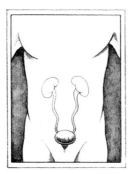

The kidneys are a pair of ear-shaped organs located above the waist, towards the back of the body.

## TRADITIONAL CHINESE INTERPRETATION

| | |
|---|---|
| Element: | Water |
| Partner organ: | Bladder |
| Climate: | Cold |
| Season: | Winter |
| Colour: | Blue/black |
| Time of day: | 5–7 p.m. |
| Body tissue: | Bones and marrow |
| Voice sound: | Moaning |
| Sense organ: | Ears |
| Reflector: | Head hair |
| Taste: | Salty |
| Emotion: | Fear |

## SYMPTOMS OF IMBALANCE

### Physical Symptoms

Premature ageing and senility • Sterility and impotence •
Poor sexual development • Retarded growth • Dark
bags under the eyes • Craving for salty foods • Broken,
split, dull hair • Oedema • Fluid-retention and bloating •
Lymphatic congestion • Lower back pain • Premature
greying of hair, loss of hair • Soft or brittle, weak bones •
Urination problems • Aversion to cold • Lethargy,
frequent yawning • Knee problems • Poor
short term memory

The Chinese believe that it is essential that we preserve our kidneys, the deepest organ in the body storing our *Jing*. *Jing* is thought to determine our constitutional make-up and govern our development, especially in the early stages of life. *Jing* is also thought to be difficult to replenish once it is depleted. *Jing* is called the 'root of life' because it is the source of reproduction, development and maturation; cases of sterility and impotence, or slow sexual maturation are kidney problems. The kidneys store reproductive energy and are very important in determining the length of our lives and our level of vitality. All sexual energy comes from the kidneys, so any sexual or reproductive dysfunction (such as impotence, frigidity or sterility) can be traced to the kidneys. Premature ageing, lethargy, lack of perception, wishy-washy behaviour and aching in the lower part of the back also reflect a lack of vital *Jing*. The entire body and all its organs need this extremely precious, inherited essence in order to thrive and survive. In Chinese medicine, the kidneys and adrenal glands are believed to contribute to the warmth of the body, our energy levels, sexual appetite, and strength in general.

Long hours working or studying can weaken the kidneys and can have a negative impact on the spleen. The body doesn't lie and the effects of tobacco, alcohol, eating on the run, lack of or excessive exercise and late nights will eventually catch up with you and could impair your health! Rest and relaxation is crucial to help strengthen the kidneys, winding down in a salt bath and having regular, early nights would make a positive difference. The reason why I have recommended a salt bath is that salt is the flavour connected to the kidneys and it is highly beneficial to have regular baths with Dead Sea salts. I find that I intuitively crave baths with these, especially if I am tired or during the Winter months. I not only feel restored and regenerated after such a bath, but deeply relaxed. Through the ages, Dead Sea salts have been known to have a very beneficial and therapeutic effect on the entire body and skin. They contain numerous minerals including potassium and magnesium, two key minerals very often deficient in today's diet. Magnesium is nature's tranquilliser and potassium helps to regulate the fluid balance in the body, which can often be adversely affected as a consequence of weakened kidney *qi*. Dead Sea salt preparations that I enjoy using include Aveda's Aqua Therapy Formula™ and Origins Ginger Salts™ that also contains the warming essential oil of ginger. Do ensure that you drink several glasses of water (preferably warm water in the Winter months) before, during and after your bath to rehydrate your body.

As mentioned, the kidneys are strongly related to sexual performance. Too much sex and frequent pregnancies can weaken the body and drain the kidney energy, thus reducing our vitality. The Chinese used to regard sex as a cause of disease; a book entitled *The Classic of the Simple Girl* (Sui Dynasty, AD 581–618) made the following recommendations on the frequency of male ejaculation.

*Male Sexual Health*

| Age | Average Health | Above Average Health |
| --- | --- | --- |
| 20 | Once a day | Twice a day |
| 30 | Every other day | Once a day |
| 40 | Every 4 days | Every 3 days |
| 50 | Every 10 days | Every 5 days |
| 60 | Every 20 days | Every 10 days |
| 70+ | Abstain! | Once a month |

Ejaculation for a man and, to a lesser extent, orgasm for a woman deplete the kidney essence.

Apart from the kidneys, the liver and heart notably contribute to a normal and happy sexual life. As the heart is also related to the kidneys, the two must support and nourish each other. Just as a kidney deficiency can weaken the heart, a heart deficiency caused by sadness and anxiety can weaken the kidneys and cause impotence or the inability to reach orgasm. The liver is responsible for the smooth flow of blood and *qi*, particularly in the lower part of the body. Stagnation here can also influence our sex life and lead to inability to reach orgasm or frigidity/impotence.

your body's own sex and energy centre

Our kidney essence is known to be depleted by the ageing process. Common symptoms in old age such as hearing difficulties, brittle bones and memory problems arise as a result of the decline of kidney essence.

※

### Emotional Symptoms

Fear • Wishy-washy behaviour • Lack of willpower •
Panic attacks • Weakness, timidity • Apprehension •
Learning difficulties • Feeling overwhelmed • Fear of
failure • Paranoid, suspicious behaviour • Complaining •
Depression

※

### Helping you understand more about the Mind–Body Link

The kidneys are known as the seat of fear, which we can see manifested when adrenaline is released in 'fight or flight' situations. When the kidneys are weakened or damaged, this may indicate that unexpressed or unacknowledged fears are building up within us. Kidney problems can therefore be related to holding on to old emotional patterns, or to negative emotions that are not being consciously released. Shock too is associated with the kidneys – this is said to explain the peculiar occurrence of people who can go grey overnight, or develop a white streak in their hair after hearing shocking news.

Willpower and ambition are governed by the Water Element. Anyone lacking willpower is expressing a symptom of a Water imbalance. However, if the energy in the kidneys is excessive, workaholism may result, as we can be driven on by a fear of failure.

Metaphysically, kidney stones have been seen as the manifestation of unshed tears or sadness. Releasing these feelings indicates a movement forward to a new state of being.

※

Fully grounding the body is important to strengthen the base and kidney energy. 'Grounding' activities include any work with the earth such as gardening, walking in the countryside, etc. Lean up against a tree and feel the strength and power it gives to you. Imagine that roots are coming out of your toes; see these roots going deep into the earth, anchoring you firmly to the ground. Feel safe and secure and allow your fears to be absorbed by the Earth and transmuted (*see Earth meditation, page 60*).

## the 9 ways to health

### way 1: chinese and natural nutrition

#### FOODS FOR THE WATER ELEMENT

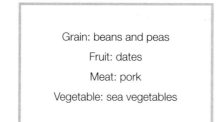

Grain: beans and peas
Fruit: dates
Meat: pork
Vegetable: sea vegetables

The taste of the Water Element (which encompasses the kidneys and the bladder) is salty, so small amounts of naturally salty foods in the diet are beneficial. However, excessive cravings for salt, or a dislike of salt, means you should keep an eye on the health of the kidneys. The salty flavour enters the kidneys and in small amounts can either nourish and support them or in excessive amounts can aggravate a Water imbalance.

The kidneys regulate the acid balance in the body and the mineral levels in the blood. All kidney problems are thought to have a strong link with acid/alkaline imbalances in the body. Ideally our acid/alkaline balance should be 80 per cent alkaline and 20 per cent acid, although in modern-day living the reverse is often true.

## DIETARY TIPS

※ As the 'cold' aggravates the Water Element and the kidneys, it is important in the winter season (and when the weather is cold and your energy is low) to favour more warming and heating methods of cooking. These include baking, roasting and grilling. A slow-cooked casserole, for example, will be more warming than a quickly cooked stir-fry.

※ Include plenty of seasonal root vegetables (preferably grown locally) in your winter diet. These are ideal in casseroles, roasted or grilled and have warming properties.

※ Have you ever noticed that your body temperature has plummeted in a situation of fear or shock? Fear is the primary emotion associated with the Water Element and gives rise to coldness on both the physical and emotional level. Whereas joy creates warmth and a free flow of energy through the body, fear creates coldness and a contraction of that flow. Comfort your body and soul through foods with warming properties (listed in the foods that strengthen section) and prepare them in line with the warming methods such as roasting, grilling or slow cooking.

### Foods that strengthen the Kidneys and Water Element
*(also see Recipes, page 285):*

※ Celery is high in organic sodium; miso (a Japanese fermented rice puree) contains salt and the lactobacteria that are so important to our health to restore the pH balance in the intestines.

※ Tamari sauce – the wheat-free version of soy sauce – is a good substitute for salt, to be used in moderation in cooking. If you do consume salt, ensure that it is sea salt.

※ Fish is also considered to be highly beneficial for the kidneys, perhaps because of seafood's connection with water and tinned salmon is particularly good for building strong bones. Oysters are particularly rich in zinc, a mineral that supports the reproductive system and have a well-earned reputation as an aphrodisiac! Other sources of zinc include sesame seeds, organic offal, red meat, eggs and pulses.

※ Aduki, black and kidney beans are rich in potassium and have a special affinity with the kidneys, possibly due to their kidney-like colour and shape.

※ Grains such as buckwheat, rice, barley and millet. Millet is alkaline and can help lower acid levels in the body. Buckwheat has warming properties and is known to heat the blood and the whole body. Wheat and rye are the most acidic of all grains and so are best avoided while you are working on raising the alkaline levels in your body.

※ Beetroot is a very cleansing food for the kidneys and bladder and is high in potassium, magnesium and vitamin A.

※ Wintertime is the best time of the year to eat meat and the Chinese recommend that foods such as bone marrow, oxtail, kidneys and red meat are added to stews. However, with the current scare over some of these foods, always search out a reputable organic farmer to ensure that the meat is safe, and free from additives and steroids.

※ Fruits of the forest such as blackberries and cranberries are excellent cleansers.

※ Increase alkaline-rich foods such as fresh fruit and vegetables and millet. Water-rich fruits such as water melons and grapes are said to help prevent kidney stones (although if you suffer from feeling the cold, consume them only in warmer months); celery, asparagus and kelp all stimulate urination.

※ Other foods to increase in your diet are walnuts, all leafy green vegetables (such as broccoli, watercress, parsley), green beans and peas, courgettes, lettuce, celery, various forms of green cabbage (such as Savoy, wintergreen), beetroot, swedes, turnips and marrows.

your body's own sex and energy centre

❋ Sea vegetables are essential to include in the diet and they are easy to assimilate as the protein is almost predigested and, coming from the sea, they have a real affinity with the Water Element. They are extremely high in minerals, and can be added to dishes to increase the nutritional value. Kombu can be put into soups and stews; adding a piece of kombu to the water and cider vinegar you soak beans and pulses in reduces the flatulence that some legumes can bestow! Wakame (tiny strips of seaweed) can be soaked for 10 minutes in water, drained and then added to a stir-fry with rice. If you use a small amount to start with, you really cannot taste it (for those who are repulsed by the thought of eating seaweed!) but you will get all those valuable minerals from including it in your diet.

❋ To ensure that you protect your bones against premature osteoporosis, it is essential that you include mineral-rich foods in your diet, especially calcium, magnesium and silica (*see pages 94 and 95 for food sources*). Solgar produce two excellent silica formulas, one called Vegetal Silica (from horsetail) and the other Oceanic Silica (from red algae).

❋ Foods that are particularly helpful in combating coldness in the body include ginger, cinnamon, nutmeg, dill and fennel seeds, lamb, chicken, trout, sweet potatoes, turnips, onion and garlic.

**Foods that weaken the Kidneys and Water Element:**

❋ Fizzy drinks (including carbonated water), wine, salt, citrus fruits and the nightshade family all disrupt the natural balance of calcium and magnesium which can result in bone loss.

❋ Reduce the amount of acid-forming foods in your diet such as coffee, tea and refined foods such as pastry, bread, biscuits, sweets and other convenience foods.

❋ The nightshade family (peppers, aubergines, tomatoes and potatoes) together with dairy products, shellfish, citrus fruits and nuts are thought to raise levels of a protein by-product called albumen, which can promote congestion in the kidneys.

When the moisture level in the body falls too low, kidney stones can develop, and this is one of the reasons why it is important to drink pure water every day (not coffee or even herbal teas, but pure water). Although the current thinking is to drink copious amounts of water, the kidneys are thought to only move six glasses of water a day (this includes liquids that are already in the body as well as what you drink), so it is important to balance the amount of fluid you consume: too much can be as bad as too little. Also, iced water is not advisable – keep it room temperature or even warmer during the Winter months.

## way 2: herbs and spices

* Cinnamon is the key spice that I have chosen for the Water Element as it has a particular affinity for the kidneys and is excellent to include in your diet. A hot tea can be made by boiling cinnamon bark for 20 minutes, or try some of the commercial teas such as Hambledon Herbs organic Spice Delight, Body Wisdom Organics, Water Element tea or Yogi tea.
* Cloves too are contained in some of the above teas and help to warm you when you suffer from low vitality or coldness due to depleted kidney *qi* and can even help to strengthen a weak back if the pain is due to low kidney energy. They can also help prevent the Winter cold bugs from getting you!
* Fresh nettles steamed or in juice form (Schoenenberger herbal juices) are extremely rich in minerals, especially iron and the plant has incredible restorative and tonic properties. It stimulates the kidneys, so helping to flush excess water and toxins out of your body due to its valuable diuretic properties.
* Saw palmetto berries have been used for hundreds of years as a general tonic for the male reproductive system. Research has shown that is it effective in treating enlarged prostate, so helping to reduce symptoms such as urinary disorders and impotence.

※ Damiana is refuted to be an aphrodisiac and is used for a lowered libido.

※ Look for herbal tincture blends (ideally organic) that include some of these herbs that have a healing affinity with the Water Element such as the Water Element Organic Herbal Elixir produced by Body Wisdom Organics.

## way 3: exercise

According to Chinese medicine, Winter is the worst time of the year for strenuous exercise; instead it is a time for conserving and replenishing energy levels. Enough exercise to get the circulation moving and to warm the body up is ideal during this season. Brisk walking and a swimming programme are suitable, as light exercises such as these are the best ways to get warm and ensure that the *qi* and blood keep moving throughout the body. T'ai Chi and Qigong are particularly good forms of exercise as they do not deplete the body of vital *qi*.

The stretch for the kidney and bladder meridian is described on *page 135.*

## way 4: massage and reflex points

Traditionally, the meridian point known as Bladder 23 can be rubbed to stimulate the kidney region and enhance energy levels. To intensify the effects, use a blend of the essential oils recommended such as the cinnamon and clove oil by Aveda while massaging this area (*see page 140*). Kidney 27 should be held or massaged as you make the sound 'WOOOOOO' and visualize a dark blue colour (*see diagram of Bladder 23, page 140, and the Kidney meridian, overleaf*) cleansing your body.

One of the main neuro-lymphatic points is situated 2 cm above your navel and 2 cm to either side (*see page 160*) which can be rubbed to strengthen the kidneys. It is even more powerful when combined with three other significant neuro-lymphatic points – the thymus (*page 75*), the spleen (*page 75*) and Kidney 27 (*page 160*).

The kidney reflex on the feet cannot be separated from those of the bladder and ureter. The bladder reflexology point is located on the inside of both feet near the heel. Trace up the tendon, which represents the urethra, until you reach the kidney reflex. Gently massage this area by 'walking' your thumb from the bladder to the kidney, feeling for any 'crystals'. (*See page 23 for massage techniques.*) As the ears are connected to the kidneys, it would be worthwhile stimulating the ear reflex found at the base of your two outer toes. As talc is often the preferred medium for reflexology, why not try the warming talc by Origins called Ginger Dust™ which is talc-free and contains oat flour, corn flour and ginger. Or make your own (*see page 73*).

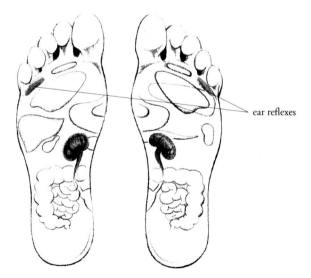

ear reflexes

*Reflexology Points for the Kidneys (shaded)*

### Healthy Hair

As the kidneys reflect the quality of lustre of our hair, preventative measures to promote a healthy head of hair are to be encouraged. While it is important to understand the internal effect of the kidneys on your hair, it is equally important to use hair care products that are both natural, gentle and nourishing to your hair and scalp. One company that I strongly believe in as well as personally use their hair products is Aveda. There are a variety of reasons why I recommend their products, which include their (genuine) company philosophy of caring for the world we live in, their excellent research and understanding of how plant-derived ingredients affect the body and mind and their goal of using the highest quality organic ingredients where possible. Many health and beauty companies with prettily packaged holistic products often fall short of their claims, but with Aveda I have always felt safe in recommending their products to my patients. That is not to say there are not other excellent hair care products on the market, just make sure you check the contents and quality of the hair treatment you are using.

An excellent way to improve the health of your hair is scalp massage as it not only increases the strength of your hair, but it can thicken it by increasing the diameter of each hair. Another benefit of scalp massage is that it relieves tension, increases the blood supply to your brain and scalp so has the advantage of making you feel more alert, and distributes our natural oil to the end of the hair. In Indian Ayurvedic medicine, sesame oil (preferably warmed gently) is used on the scalp and you could add a few drops of lavender if you need calming or for oily hair, rosemary if you need a lift. Leave on for up to an hour after massage and keep wrapped in cling film with a towel over to keep the heat in. If you need relaxing, an excellent product to try is Calming Composition™ by Aveda which contains clarified jojoba oil, rose and other plant and flower essences or Dr Haushka Neem Hair oil which can be massaged into your scalp for a treatment.

In folk medicine, drinking sage tea was thought to encourage the growth of thick and healthy hair (do not use if pregnant) and I certainly believe in the benefit of drinking nettle tea to improve the quality of your hair. For extra shine, try rinsing your hair with nettle tea that has been steeped, strained and cooled; for dark hair, adding a teaspoon of vinegar to your final rinse can make your hair shine more, just as rosemary too is used as a scalp stimulant to add shine to dark hair, but I found it left my hair slightly dull, so I would advise leaving the rosemary on for 20 minutes before washing your hair. Aveda do an organic shampoo and conditioner containing Rosemary and Mint which is a very refreshing and stimulating product to use. The calming herb chamomile is traditionally used as a rinse to lighten and brighten blonde or fair hair. Use a good chamomile shampoo and conditioner which is rich in natural plant extracts (my favourite is Aveda's Chamomile shampoo and colour conditioner which revitalizes the colour naturally while giving absolutely suberb shine and softness). I also use the Personal Blends in a conditioning formula so I can choose a perfect honey colour but it then has my favourite Aveda Key Element™ pure plant aromas to balance my constitution according to the Ayurvedic system. For those of you who like to use a more permanent colour on your hair or wish to cover grey, do remember that some dyes can be very harsh on your hair. Full Spectrum (Aveda) plant technology uses essential oils to create a new colour development process that is 97% naturally derived and protects your hair.

## way 5: acupressure

The kidney meridian actually begins on the sole of the foot and travels up the inside ankle to the inner thigh. It then goes within and connects to both the kidney and bladder before running back to the surface where it travels up the front of the body and finishes at the base of the collar bone – Kidney 27 (see *diagram overleaf*). Kidney 27 is an important acupressure point to massage if you are feeling run down as it can help to correct the energy flow in your body, energize and increase alertness. Kidney 1 on your feet, called the *wellspring of life* points are also powerful points to hold or massage.

To trace the meridian, start from kidney 1 on your feet, run your palms up the inside of each foot to your inner ankle and circle around it.

Let your hand travel up the front of your body to kidney 27 and on reaching these points, massage to stimulate your *qi*.

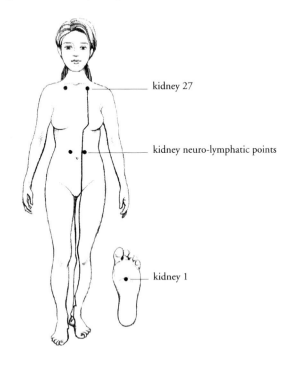

*The Kidney Meridian and Acupuncture Points*

### Kidney 3

Kidney 3 is located on the inside of the ankle, halfway between the Achilles tendon and the ankle bone. This point enhances the energy of the kidneys and also can help to strengthen willpower, thus restoring both courage and self-confidence.

### Kidney 6

Kidney 6 is located near Kidney 3 and is one finger-width directly beneath the inside of the ankle bone in a little hollow. It can be sensitive to pressure, so apply it with care. This point helps to balance the Water Element and the emotions that correspond to it (such as fear and depression). It also supports the lungs by opening the chest and can calm the mind. For both Kidney 3 and Kidney 6, hold your heel with one hand and gently stimulate the acupressure point by rubbing it with the thumb of your other hand in a circular motion. Do be gentle with this area and never use too much pressure.

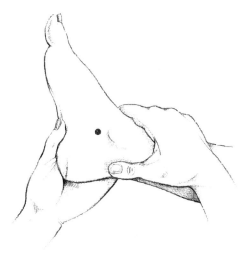

*Kidney 3 (under the right thumb) and 6 (above) Acupressure Points*

These two points along with Bladder 23 would greatly benefit from moxibustion (*see 'Taking a Deeper Look at Chinese Medicine'*) when there are symptoms of fatigue, weakness and cold.

It is important to protect the kidney area. The Japanese used to do this by wearing a *harikame* – a band worn around the hara area to support the immune system and keep the body healthy and strong. You can make your own version by tying a scarf around your waist. Ensure that the scarf is approximately 16 cm wide at the back, and covers you 8 cm above and below the waist. It will also keep you very warm in bed, allowing you to wake feeling more refreshed and rested.

# way 6: essential oils

**Cedarwood:** strengthens the energy of the kidneys, has an affinity for the genito-urinary system and is good for bladder infections. Gives extra strength on an emotional level during difficult times, helping to transform these periods into opportunities to learn and gain spiritual insight and wisdom. *Strength factor: Weak*

**Cypress:** detoxifies and decongests the body, helping to restore balance and equilibrium to the acid/alkali levels. Helps with hidden fears or fears of unknown origin. Added to the bath (4–6 drops along with the same amount of the Bach flower remedy Aspen), it can soothe away such fears. Also helpful for depression associated with being oppressed by another. *Strength factor: Medium*

**Fennel:** has an affinity for the kidneys and, by strengthening the kidney *yang* energy, plays a supportive role to the spleen. *Strength factor: Strong*

**Geranium:** helps on an emotional level to balance willpower when we feel unable to contain and control our personal ambition to succeed. Helps to bring out the qualities needed to soften and slow this driving force. Gently supports energy and calms the mind. Excellent for hormonal imbalance and lymphatic congestion. *Strength factor: Strong*

**Ginger:** strengthens energy and fire, helping to activate willpower when we are apathetic or procrastinating; stimulates inspiration and creativity. Can help to rekindle the flames of passion when they have been dampened by an imbalance in the Water Element! *Strength factor: Medium*

**Juniper:** an excellent diuretic, helping to flush out excess water from the system. A decongestant, eliminating toxins and stimulating the lymphatic system. Helps to combat infections, especially in the genito-urinary system. A warming and stimulating oil that warms cold hands and lifts fatigue. Uplifts and inspires those who have allowed negativity and fear to consume their thoughts and control their actions. Drives away the fear of failure connected to self-doubt and insecurity, restoring resolve and determination. *Strength factor: Medium*

**Thyme:** adds warmth to the kidneys and helps us to overcome fears that arise from a known cause. Instils courage and boosts low morale by replacing poor self-esteem and apathy with vigour, confidence and drive. *Strength factor: Strong*

**Rosemary:** raises low self-esteem and encourages optimism and confidence. A supreme memory stimulant. *Strength factor: Strong*

An excellent blend to massage on your lower back and Bladder 23 point (*see page 140*) is the Cinnamon Bark and Clove Oil by Aveda in their Singular Notes range which is excellent for tiredness and the oils can help to strengthen a weak back (which can be triggered by low kidney energy). Both are excellent essential oils for warming the kidneys when you feel tired, shivery and cold in the Winter months but need to be purchased in a professionally blended formula as they are strong oils which need to be used with caution. Clove and Cinnamon are also found in the Water Element Organic Essential Oil Blend by Body Wisdom Organics along with Geranium and Cedarwood.

**N.B.** All essential oils should be used with care and true kidney ailments need prompt medical attention and proper diagnosis.

## way 7: flower remedies

**Aspen:** for vague fears and apprehensions and unconscious fears when you cannot understand where the feelings are coming from. Often people who need Aspen are sensitive to psychic influences – children who need the light on at night because they are scared of ghosts benefit from Aspen. A glass of water with 2–4 drops of this remedy left beside the bed at night will help children who wake with nightmares.

**Mimulus:** for tangible fears that arise in everyday life. Those who need Mimulus are often sensitive souls with a delicate constitution, which ties in with the kidney type of personality, who has to be careful not to burn the candle at both ends.

**Olive:** Exhaustion is felt both mentally and physically when our kidney *qi* is depleted. Olive restores strength and vitality to body and soul.

**Rock Rose:** the remedy for extreme, acute fears that border on terror. For those almost frozen into a state of fear; children who wake screaming after a particularly bad nightmare should be given this remedy in the same way as Aspen.

**Star of Bethlehem:** the remedy for trauma and shock, which have a profound affect on the state of the kidneys. Soothes and comforts, restoring the body's self-healing mechanism and heralding the return of calm.

**Evening Primrose:** FF13 is the primary remedy to support kidney and adrenal function and is used when the kidneys do not efficiently filter and clear water from the body.

**Camellia:** FF3 activates the rear pituitary that supports the kidneys, enabling them to regulate the fluids of the body.

**Arum Lily:** FF17 is the flower formula for the reproductive system that the kidney supports, and so is helpful for infertility, impotence, frigidity etc.

**Anemone:** FF20 supports our structure and bones, which are directly linked, according to traditional Chinese medicine, to the Kidneys and the Water Element.

Alternatively, try the Phytobiophysics Kidney Meridian Formula or the Water Element Flower Formula by Body Wisdom Organics which contains a blend of flowers including the Bladder and Kidney meridian essences.

*You may also find some appropriate flower remedies for supporting the Water Element in the chapter on the Bladder (page 141).*

## way 8: affirmations

- ❈ My kidneys cleanse and care for my body.
- ❈ I allow the *qi* to regenerate in my kidneys, replenishing the very core of my being.
- ❈ I am safe and secure and able to face any challenges that may arise.
- ❈ My willpower is resolute and gives me newfound strength.
- ❈ I cherish my kidneys as they are the root of all life and new beginnings.

*See also the Bladder chapter, page 142, for affirmations that may be used in conjunction with these.*

## way 9: meditation for the water element

*See Bladder chapter, page 142.*

# understanding the wood element

The key to

- ❉ Detoxifying your Body
- ❉ Improving your Eyesight
- ❉ Strengthening your Nails
- ❉ Relieving Headaches and Nausea
- ❉ Resolving Frustration and Anger

**Partner Organs:** Liver and gallbladder, which have a very close relation-ship not only in the Chinese system, but also in Western medicine. For example, the liver as seen in Western pathology produces bile, which is then stored and concentrated in the gallbladder.

**Climate:** Wind. It is essential to protect your body from the wind, the most vulnerable area being the back of the neck and shoulders. Springtime colds and flus can be greatly reduced by following the simple advice of wearing a scarf. The liver is also susceptible to *internal wind* in the body (not flatulence!), which can give rise to stiffness, numbness, convulsions, twitches, pains that move in the body and clumsiness.

**Season:** The Wood Element is linked to Spring, the time of year when the earth begins to burst alive with energy and new growth. The growth of plants can mirror how the body energy changes with the seasons. The body's energy rises and moves from within to the surface in Spring; plants, too, begin to grow above the ground, their growth upward and outward.

**Colour:** Green is the colour of the Wood Element – interestingly the colour associated with jealousy and revenge, the emotions linked to the gallbladder. An obsession with or an aversion to this colour can point to an imbalance in the Wood Element. Chinese practitioners with a trained eye will notice a green tinge on the face, a viable diagnostic indication of imbalance.

**Time of day:** The time the gallbladder is in power, according to the Chinese body clock, is 11 p.m.–1 a.m. The liver follows on from 1–3 a.m. Failing to sleep, or waking between these times, can point to an imbalance in the liver or gallbladder. This element also has an influence on the quality and length of sleep, and can induce dreams of trials, fights and suicide according to ancient Chinese texts. It is important to be in bed before this element comes into power as the liver is involved in filtering the blood. To do this effectively, the body needs to be horizontal because when you are up and about, the liver directs blood to the parts of the body needing it. If, for example, you are exercising, the blood is sent to nourish the muscles. Ideally you should aim to be in bed before 11 p.m., otherwise the liver energy is diverted from its important physical function of cleaning and renewing the blood. Waking unrefreshed and tired in the morning can show that the liver has not purified the blood efficiently. Excess artificial light, working for long hours or shift work through the night can also prevent the liver from regenerating effectively.

**Body Tissue:** The Wood Element controls the tendons and ligaments and the way in which these interact with the muscles. If the liver has not cleansed the blood sufficiently or if there is a deficiency of blood, the tendons will suffer from malnutrition – giving rise to stiffness, difficulty flexing and extending the joints, numbness and spasms. Therefore, for any diseases that involve the tendons we must look at the Wood Element.

**Voice sound:** Shouting – a very obvious connection as the emotion of the liver, anger, frequently manifests as emotional outbursts and raging arguments as the pressure cooker lid finally blows off! Someone with a loud voice is also demonstrating 'liverish' tendencies.

**Sense Organ:** The Wood Element nourishes the eyes (with the gall bladder). The health of the eyes is seen as being dependent on the health of the liver, so any visual disturbances can be interpreted as a reflection of the state of your liver. If a problem occurs in the liver, the eyes can suffer from dryness, redness, night blindness, 'floaters' (black spots before the eyes), cataracts, glaucoma or blurred vision.

**Reflector:** The nails are considered an extension of the tendons, so problems such as changes in nail colour, brittle nails, ridges on the nails or weak, splitting nails all tell us that something about the Wood Element is being imbalanced.

**Symptoms of Imbalance:** The liver is the key organ associated with the Wood Element. A healthy liver is like a tender young tree that is green and flexible, yet firmly rooted into the earth. The sap is fresh and vital like the blood in our body when it is clean and pure. As it bends in the wind, its movements are graceful and fluid, just like our body when in balance, with energy flowing smoothly and effortlessly. When the liver energy stagnates, however, we can become brittle, wooden and inflexible in both body and mind. Symptoms of imbalance include migraines, headaches, stiffness and tension in the neck and shoulder area, nausea, vomiting, premenstrual syndrome, vision disturbances, weak and flaky nails. Emotional imbalances include rage, anger, frustration, bitterness, jealousy and indecision.

# your body's own fat buster

## what your gall bladder does for you

Here is another important organ that does not mind staying behind the scenes. This supportive organ assists the liver and the small intestine in breaking up fats. Keep an eye out for the following physical symptoms which include headaches, pain on the right side of trunk and weak, splitting nails as well as emotional symptoms from Chinese medicine that include jealousy, resentment and aggressive behaviour.

### TRADITIONAL WESTERN UNDERSTANDING

The gall bladder cooperates with the liver, which makes about 2 litres a day of a liquid called bile which is concentrated and stored in the gall bladder. Bile acts like a washing-up powder, breaking up fats in the food.

When food enters the small intestine, a hormone is released which instructs the gall bladder to contract and send bile directly to the small intestine to assist in breaking down fatty foods. Salts in the bile help the body absorb fat-soluble vitamins. Synthetic drugs, together with natural hormones and steroids, are excreted in the bile. The bile is then sent back to the liver to be recycled, and so the process turns full circle. Bile is, in addition, a good laxative which ensures that peristalsis (movement of the large intestines) takes place.

Gallstones affect about 15 per cent of the population. They form when cholesterol levels rise. Steroids and the contraceptive pill predispose us to gallstones, so does too much fat and protein in the diet – ironically, too little fat and skipping meals are also contributory factors. Eating a meal which contains a little fat, preferably essential fatty acids or olive oil, will stimulate the gall bladder into releasing bile. Low bile levels can result in an overgrowth of bacteria in the small intestine, leading to fermentation of the foods and bloating.

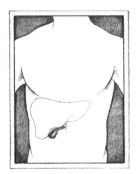

The gall bladder is a pear-shaped organ the size of your thumb, situated underneath the liver.

**TRADITIONAL CHINESE INTERPRETATION**

| | |
|---|---|
| Element: | Wood |
| Partner organ: | Liver |
| Climate: | Wind |
| Season: | Spring |
| Colour: | Green |
| Time of day: | 11 p.m.–1 a.m. |
| Body tissue: | Tendons/ligaments |

nine ways to body wisdom

172

| | |
|---|---|
| Voice sound: | Shouting |
| Sense organ: | Eyes |
| Reflector: | Nails |
| Taste: | Sour |
| Emotion: | Anger |

## SYMPTOMS OF IMBALANCE

### Physical Symptoms

Pain on right side of trunk • Migraines and headaches •
Stiff shoulders and neck area • Weak, splitting nails •
Difficulty digesting fatty foods • Bitter taste in mouth •
Pale stools

In Chinese medicine the gall bladder and liver are affected by anger, frustration and bottled-up resentment. We all know expressions such as 'she had the gall to accuse me' and other references to people being 'liverish'. Irritability, thirst, headaches and a bitter taste in the mouth can point to gall bladder trouble. Stagnation of energy in the body can harm the spleen, and symptoms of imbalance such as oedema and lethargy may become apparent. Excess damp in the body leads it to try to create more heat in an attempt to 'dry' the damp, bringing another set of problems known as 'damp heat'. This often occurs in the pelvis; vaginal infections, thrush, fibroids and other genital problems can manifest as a result.

✳

### Emotional Symptoms

Jealousy • Resentment • Aggressive behaviour •<br>Indecision • Frustration • Unexpressed anger •<br>Bitterness

✳

### Helping you understand more about the Mind–Body Link

In Chinese medicine the gall bladder and liver are affected by anger, frustration and bottled-up resentment. These feelings deplete our energy levels and can lead to long term health problems.

The Chinese believe anger in short explosive bursts is actually healthy, but in our society, especially for women, this is often deemed unacceptable. Seeing a counsellor or even talking to a close friend to get feelings out and free the body of emotional pain must be a priority. Try releasing pent-up emotions by punching the air or a pillow, or do what the Native American tribespeople do: the 'power stomp'. If you have a drum, play the drum too! Shake your hands to release any stress held within as if you were shaking it out of your body. Punch the air to get it all out. Stamp your feet and make the sound 'Ho', allowing it to come from deep within, not just your throat. If you are angry with someone or something, let your feelings out in this safe way, rather than keeping them inside bubbling away until you finally explode! Once you have physically begun to release the anger within, it is ideal to follow with the Wood meditation – Resolving Anger, to help soothe and heal your body, emotions and soul.

The Chinese believe that when the gall bladder is working efficiently, its owner will be able to take clear and decisive action. They have an expression for this: 'Big Gall bladder' (meaning courageous). When the Wood Element is healthy, we are graceful and flexible both physically and

✳

mentally. Our powers of judgement and decision-making are sound, our vision clear and our actions resolute.

# the 9 ways to health

## way 1: chinese and natural nutrition

### FOODS FOR THE WOOD ELEMENT

> Grain: wheat
>
> Fruit: peach
>
> Meat: chicken
>
> Vegetable: leak

### DIETARY TIPS

1. Excessive fasting or skipping meals, in particular breakfast, can encourage the formation of gallstones.
2. Eating smaller and more frequent meals helps to prevent a concentration of bile in the gall bladder.

**Foods that strengthen the Gall Bladder and Wood Element**
*(also see Recipes, page 286):*

The taste for the Wood Element is sour, so craving a lot of sour foods, e.g., lemons, sauerkraut and pickled snacks, can be feeding a Wood imbalance, or an indication that the body is trying to correct one. The body knows what it needs to strengthen itself.

❋ Foods that are supportive to the gall bladder include artichokes, green beans, beetroot, carrots, dandelions, endive, fennel, lemon, kale, mustard greens, nettles, olive oil, parsley, radish, sweet potato and watercress.

❋ Soya bean protein (organic), nuts, beans, lentils, peas and lima beans help prevent gallstones.

❋ In Greece, where olive oil is consumed regularly, gallstones are relatively unknown. Vegetarians too have fewer gallstones than the average person, probably due to the higher levels of vitamin C and fibre in their diets.

❋ A small quantity of alcohol (half a glass of wine or beer) can increase the breakdown of cholesterol, making less of it available to produce gallstones.

❋ Choosing oat bran porridge for breakfast could help to lower your cholesterol levels by up to 10%.

❋ Protect your gall bladder and lower your cholesterol levels by supplementing your diet with lecithin, a well-known fat emulsifier. It has a detergent action that helps break up cholesterol in the body. Simply sprinkle on food. Also ensure that you include essential fatty acids in your diet.

❋ Dandelions are an excellent natural source of lecithin and make an interesting addition to your salad.

❋ The B-complex vitamins (found in whole grain foods) help the gall bladder to empty more efficiently.

**Foods that weaken the Gall Bladder and Wood Element**

❋ Certain foods have a negative effect on the gall bladder particularly greasy, fried foods high in cholesterol.

❋ Excessive amounts of alcohol have a negative impact on both the liver and the gall bladder.

❋ The body needs at least 5 to 10 grams of fat in one meal each day to stimulate the gall bladder to release bile and when our fat intake is drastically cut, the gall bladder does not contract to expel bile, leading to the possible formation of gallstones. Do ensure that you eat the kind of fats such as raw olive oil, essential fatty acids (*page 16*) and oily fish.

*See the Liver chapter, page 193, for further information about foods for the Wood Element.*

## way 2: herbs and spices

* ❋ An ancient herbal remedy for gall bladder problems is black radish. When the bile duct becomes obstructed, inflammation can occur. This magnesium-rich herb can help alleviate and soothe this condition and is useful in the treatment of gallstones. It is available in juice form through Schoenenberger.
* ❋ Other herbs that have been used to give relief to gall bladder problems are equal parts of fennel seed, wild yam root and Oregon grape root.
* ❋ Try cooking using turmeric, an Indian spice that is excellent for both the liver and gall bladder.

*See the Liver chapter (page 198) for additional herbs and spices to aid the Wood Element.*

## way 3: exercise

Exercise that helps us to release stored-up frustrations and tensions also helps to reduce stagnation in the liver and gall bladder. Do ensure, however, that exercise does not become excessive or depleting. Gentle movement and stretching exercises such as T'ai Chi and yoga encourage flexibility (important for the Wood Element as it is prone to tension and stiffness). If you feel rigor mortis setting in, loosen up those muscles by simply swinging your arms and legs gently to improve circulation.

The stretch for the gall bladder and liver meridians involves sitting on the floor with your legs as wide apart as possible. Ensure that your back is straight. Put your hands together, stretch your arms over your head and take a deep breath. Exhale slowly as you stretch forward gently towards your right foot or calf – aim to reach for your toes. Go as far as your body can manage, never over-stretch. Instead, relax into a comfortable stretch and take some deep breaths. Visualize a white light flowing into the meridians and your muscles; see the congestion melting away. You should feel the stretch along the outside of your right leg and the inside of your left. Repeat twice then slowly bring your body back into an upright position. Repeat on the left side. Remember that it may take many weeks or months to achieve this. Always work at your own pace and ensure that you have warmed the muscles in your body for 10 minutes prior to stretching. If possible, join a local yoga class where you can be guided and personally instructed.

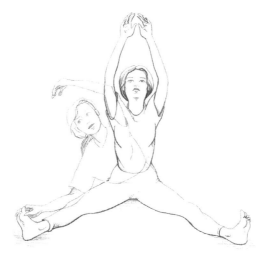

*The Gall Bladder/Liver Stretch*

## way 4: massage and reflex points

The neuro-lymphatic reflex points to stimulate gall bladder function are to be found between your 3rd and 4th ribs and your 4th and 5th ribs near your sternum. Rub firmly or tap for a minute.

The reflex point for the gall bladder is situated on the right foot, just beneath the liver reflex. Gently massage by walking your thumb over this area, feeling for any hard, granular lumps. Finish by massaging the foot with a base oil to which some essential oils have been added. *(See page 23 for massage technique and page 182 for recommended oils.)*

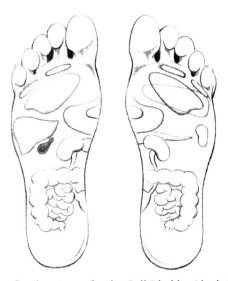

*Reflexology Point for the Gall Bladder (shaded)*

Regular massage is ideal to soften stiff muscles. As the Wood Element is responsible for the smooth flow of *qi* in the body, soothing an imbalance will focus on easing inner tension and frustration. If this tension accumulates and goes inward, then depression can result which will benefit from specific oils that help to break up stagnant emotions such as unexpressed anger or resentment *(see Essential Oils, page 182).*

## way 5: acupressure

The gall bladder meridian (*see below*) is the longest in the body. Its pathway begins at the outer corner of either eye and zigzags around the head, running down the back of the head and neck into the shoulders, round the rib cage, into the buttocks, and down the outside of the leg, finishing at the nail of the fourth toe.

To trace this meridian place the palms of both hands on the outer edge of your eyebrows, trace down towards your ears, back up to your forehead and around the back of your ears. Sweep back up and towards your forehead, over your crown, down the back of your neck and shoulders. Now, bring your hands forward and place again on your shoulders, drop them down your chest and zig zag down the side of your body, sweep them down the outside of your legs and off the fourth toes. As this is a complicated meridian, it is worthwhile carefully studying the diagram on page 000 before embarking on this exercise.

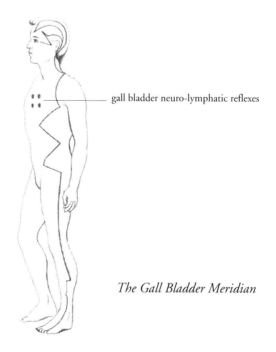

gall bladder neuro-lymphatic reflexes

*The Gall Bladder Meridian*

### Gall Bladder 20

This is at the back of the head, located between the base of the skull and the neck muscles in a little hollow of the spinal column. This point has an impact on the entire body and can relieve tension in the head and neck and improve circulation to the face and eyes. It will often be sensitive to the touch if there is congestion in these areas. It also helps with dizziness and insomnia and it can soothe and calm the nerves.

### Gall Bladder 21

This is found at the top of the shoulders, located on the big muscle at the base of the neck. It is easy to find as it is often very tight and sore! This is a classic area for reflecting our state of tension and disharmony. Massaging it eases stiffness in the neck and can also relieve pain in the shoulders and upper back.

These two points have traditionally been used to release headaches, ease fatigue and help with nervous disorders; they also have a connection with the sexual organs (so do **not** work on either point if you are pregnant).

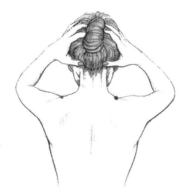

*Gall Bladder 20 (under thumbs) and 21 (on shoulders) Acupressure Points*

## way 6: essential oils

**Bergamot:** regulates and smoothes liver *qi*, encouraging an even flow of energy around the body. Calms and regulates the nervous system, nervous tension often being created by *qi* stagnation. Alleviates and releases any bottled-up resentment and frustration. *Strength factor: Medium*

**Bitter orange:** unblocks stagnant *qi* in the liver, gall bladder, stomach and intestines. Helps with emotional tension, insomnia and nauseous headaches or migraines. Ideal for abdominal distension and flatulence, indigestion, nausea, vomiting and constipation. Stimulates the gall bladder and encourages the flow of bile. *Strength factor: Medium*

**Chamomile:** eases resentment, frustration and depression that result from energy stagnating in the Wood Element. Has an impact on the solar plexus (our nerve centre) so is extremely helpful for nervous tension of either mental and physical origin. *Strength factor: Strong*

**Lavender:** cools and calms, taking the heat out of unexpressed anger that can manifest as inner rage, frustration, resentment and general irritability. Encourages the movement and flow of *qi*, releasing pent-up energy. *Strength factor: Weak*

**Mandarin:** is a mild oil that has a stimulant effect on both the liver and gall bladder. It helps the body break down fats efficiently and aids in the secretion of bile. Useful for digestive problems such as gas and can also help release pent-up emotions that can be experienced by women in the premenstrual phase of the month. *Strength factor: Weak*

Other oils of benefit include **Peppermint** and **Rosemary**. An excellent product to use for headaches and on gall bladder 20 and 21 is Peace of Mind™ by Origins which contains peppermint. It cools and refreshes, releasing congestion and stagnation in these points.

# way 7: flower remedies

**Beech:** for a tense, stiff body and a critical, irritable, dissatisfied mind. Loosens and relaxes the rigidity that encompasses both mind and body and fosters tolerance and compassion.

**Holly:** for aggressive emotions such as jealousy, envy, frustration and pent-up anger as well as outright rage, hatred and distrust which we find difficult to hold inside. Helps to transmute these emotions into their opposite: compassion and love.

**Scleranthus:** for indecision, affording clarity and allowing for decisive action to be taken. Helps with restlessness, fluctuating moods and changeable symptoms – physical and emotional ones. Focuses the mind and restores harmony and inner balance.

**Wild Oat:** helps to give direction and a sense of purpose at times when we feel vague and undecided.

**Willow:** for resentment and bitterness; for those who bear a grudge and blame others rather than accepting personal responsibility. Helps us to accept our negative emotions and take responsibility for our actions. Encourages faith, calm and optimism.

**Dandelion:** FF12 is a powerful detoxification formula that enables the body to produce healthy bile and emotionally helps to release suppressed anger and frustration especially when combined with the supporting Orchid formula (FF7).

Alternatively, try the Phytobiophysics Gall Bladder Meridian Formula or the Wood Element Flower Formula™ by Body Wisdom Organics.

You will also find some appropriate flower remedies for supporting the Wood Element in the chapter on the liver (*page 206*).

## way 8: affirmations

⁑  My gall bladder efficiently performs its function, so assisting and supporting the process of digestion.

⁑  I am able to use my powers of judgement to take clear and decisive action in my life.

⁑  I have the courage to let any repressed emotions now release in a positive and constructive manner.

*See also the Liver chapter, page 207, for affirmations that may be used in conjunction with these.*

## way 9: meditation for soul nourishment ... resolving anger

Before beginning this meditation, familiarize yourself with the diagrams of the relevant meridians (i.e., for the gall bladder and liver).

Visualize yourself nestling between two roots of a magnificent beech tree in a beautiful woodland glade where golden shafts of light filter through the lime green leaves. The sunlight catches the rich olive green of new moss on the tree trunk; there is an iridescent green light, and an air of stillness and peace. Notice the new growth of the leaf buds bursting open on slender young saplings that gently sway in the breeze. A healthy liver is compared in Chinese medicine to the tender young tree that is flexible yet firmly rooted into the earth. The sap is fresh and vital like the blood in our body when it is clean and pure. As the young sapling bends in the wind, its movements are graceful and fluid, just like your body when in balance, with the energy flowing smoothly and effortlessly around the body. The atmosphere is charged with the energy and expectancy of new life, so inspiring feelings of hope, and new beginnings. Feel the vibrant green colour that surrounds you, embracing and soothing your soul. Allow peace and tranquillity to envelop your mind, body and spirit.

Imagine your feet on the velvet green carpet of new grass beneath you – start to absorb the fresh green colour into your feet and begin to focus your energy on your big toe where the liver meridian begins. Visualize the green energy running up your foot and allow it to flow upwards on the inside of your leg, around the genitals and all the way to the right side of your ribcage where your liver and gall bladder can be found. Begin to intensify the fresh Spring green colour around these two organs and feel the green seeping into the liver and being absorbed by the gall bladder. Intensify the energy and feel it strengthening and supporting these vital organs enabling them to detoxify the body and mind more efficiently of negative emotions and physical toxins. Does your body or mind feel inflexible, rigid, stiff and wooden like an old wizened tree? Do you have problems with your eyes or weak, flaking nails? If so, this reflects that the liver energy is not flowing as it should be and is in need of some care and attention! The liver is also known as the seat of anger and is the area of the body where irritation, frustration and even rage can reside. Begin to focus inwards and tune into your liver – can you feel any anger held within? Is it from a recent event or can you feel anger from the past where you were unable to express this so the emotion was suppressed? Can you find for-giveness in your heart to release this old hurt and unresolved anger? To forgive those responsible for inflicting such pain? It is only eating away inside you and hurting you still, lowering your energy and reducing your enjoyment of life. Let it go and live life! Take a deep breath and intensify the green energy. Feel the colour enveloping your liver and gall bladder and very slowly dissolving your anger. Feel it melting and reducing in both size and importance as the cooling and refreshing green mist soothes and calms your liver. Watch as you see it evaporate and disappear in the mist. Take a few moments to finally reflect and release. You may need to repeat this meditation several times to truly let go of some anger and know that you will process it in your own time. But as you let go of the old negative emotions, know that you are allowing space for new and positive experiences to enter your life.

Now, focus this green energy at the outer corner of your eye where the gall bladder meridian begins. Send the *qi* across and down the back of the head to the base of the skull. There is a very important acupressure point which is found between the base of your skull and the neck muscles in a little hollow on either side of the spinal column. Increase the energy here and feel it relieve tension in your head, calm your nerves, soothe your eyes and dissolve any further blockages, congestion and pain held in this area. Now allow the green light to flow from your neck into the shoulders. Feel it melting and releasing any tension in these muscles, mentally feel your shoulders drop – sigh a sigh of relief as you let your burdens go that have been weighing heavily on your shoulders. Allow the green light to continue travelling down to your ribcage where your gall bladder lives. Reflect here and see if you can sense any unresolved grudges or resentment stored in your gall bladder. Allow a soft green colour to be absorbed by your gall bladder and feel this dissolving any hatred and negativity. Let the negative energy seep out of the organ and see it running through the gall bladder meridian down the side of the legs until it reaches the fourth toe where the meridian ends. Here allow it to flow out of the toe and into the earth where the negativity is transmuted. Give thanks to the Earth for this. Feel your body energized and clear. Feel the surge of this Spring energy inspiring and encouraging you to make a fresh start.

If you wish to sleep now, stay in this deeply relaxed state of being and know that you will wake in the morning feeling refreshed and rejuvenated. If however, you want to wake, then in your own time, sense your energy becoming stronger and begin to move your fingers and toes. Take a deep breath in and feel new life and energy enter your body. Open your eyes and stretch your body out feeling yourself becoming more alive, awake and full of the joys of Spring!

# your body's own detoxifier

## what your liver does for you

Considering the harmful build-up of toxins in our environment, our liver must be working double overtime! The liver is not only a detoxifier, but also stores blood, supplies more energy and produces bile to help with digestion and absorbing fats. Physical symptoms to be aware of include nausea, constipation, PMS, bloating and emotional symptoms include anger, irritability and moodiness.

### TRADITIONAL WESTERN UNDERSTANDING

The liver weighs about 1.5 kg, it is reddish-brown in colour and has two main lobes, the right lobe being six times larger than the left. It was once believed that the extent of one's health and vitality could be determined to a large degree by the health of the liver. This vital organ carries out over 500 different functions and can even regenerate its own tissue. If 90 per cent of a person's liver were removed, the remaining 10 per cent could regenerate into a complete organ!

The liver stores large quantities of nutrient-rich blood containing valuable minerals and vitamins. All the blood from the stomach and the intestines passes through the liver, allowing for full and proper absorption of nutrients. Like the spleen, the liver is an essential reservoir of the body's blood which it can release in emergencies.

The liver absorbs and stores fats, carbohydrates and proteins from our food which are then used for energy or storage in the body as fatty deposits. The liver can assist the body if it needs more immediate energy by converting stored glycogen into glucose, a simple sugar. This is sent directly into the bloodstream, to meet the body's immediate demands and keep blood sugar levels constant. Proteins are broken down and converted into their smaller components, amino acids (the nitrogenous portion not needed for new amino acids is eliminated from the body as urea).

The liver produces bile, a greenish-yellow liquid that is stored and concentrated in the gall bladder. Bile helps with the digestion and absorption of fats and stimulates the wave-like contractions called peristalsis in the large intestine. Insufficient bile can therefore contribute to constipation and digestive problems.

One of the liver's most important roles is detoxification, as it filters over a litre of blood every minute, clearing poisons, chemicals and drugs from the body and breaking these down into less toxic compounds to be easily eliminated. If the toxic load gets too high, various functions of the liver can become impaired and this can give rise to a multitude of symptoms including allergic reactions. Some classic diseases involving the liver include cirrhosis and gout, which are often caused by excessive alcohol consumption. Bruising is a sign that the liver is weak and unable to produce enough clotting factor (prothrombin). Nausea, vomiting and biliousness are other symptoms of a damaged liver, which can in turn lead to migraine. Haemorrhoids are linked with the liver: by treating this organ as well as ensuring that the bowels move regularly, haemorrhoids will often be a thing of the past.

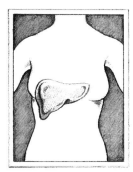

The liver is a wedge-shaped organ situated on the right-hand side of the body beneath the diaphragm and right lung.

## TRADITIONAL CHINESE INTERPRETATION

| | |
|---|---|
| Element: | Wood |
| Partner organ: | Gall Bladder |
| Climate: | Wind |
| Season: | Spring |
| Colour: | Green |
| Time of day: | 1–3 a.m. |
| Body tissue: | Tendons/ligaments |
| Voice sound: | Shouting |
| Sense organ: | Eyes |
| Reflector: | Nails |
| Taste: | Sour |
| Emotion: | Anger |

## SYMPTOMS OF IMBALANCE

### Physical Symptoms

Nausea, vomiting • Nauseous headaches, migraines • Abdominal distension, bloating • PMS, breast tenderness • Irregular, painful periods •

your body's own detoxifier

Blurred, weak vision • Spots in front of eyes • Stiff neck, shoulders, body, muscles • Haemorrhoids • Bruising • Indigestion • Flatulence, constipation • Weak nails • Aversion to wind

✳

In Chinese medicine the liver is one of the most important organs. Its key functions are seen as storing blood and ensuring the smooth flow of energy around the mind and body. When the body is at rest, the liver stores the blood and regulates the amount of blood in circulation; an inability to store and release blood contributes to stagnation of *qi* in the body. When there is a disruption of this flow of energy, many symptoms can manifest which can increase levels of both physical and mental tension within the body.

Gynaecological problems such as PMS and menstrual difficulties are linked with the liver: the meridian encircles the genital region of the body and breast tenderness can also occur if there is congestion in the liver meridian, as its pathway runs through the breasts. Lumps in the breasts and groin area can arise when there is liver stagnation. Excessive muscular tension, especially around the shoulders and neck area, is another common symptom of liver problems.

The liver can become swollen or expanded if the diet contains too many saturated fats or too much alcohol. As the organ swells, it pushes against the muscles and vertebrae, which can cause the spine to go out of alignment. Due to the relationship that the spinal nerves have to the organs, a possible cause of backache can be an imbalance in the internal organs, especially the liver, gall bladder, heart, spleen or kidneys. Backache indicating a liver imbalance is likely to be felt in the middle part of the back.

✳

## Emotional Symptoms

Anger • Irritability • Emotional repression • Depression •
Inability to plan or organize • Over-fastidious planning •
Impatience • Frustration • Moodiness • Rigid attitude •
Negative outlook • Aggression, shouting •
Nervous tension

### Helping you understand more about the Mind–Body Link

Anger is the emotion connected to the liver – not surprisingly, the sound associated with the liver is shouting. One of the biochemical jobs of the liver is to absorb nutrients from the blood and store them. Emotionally, it is thought to play a similar role, as it is believed to 'absorb anger', preventing us from becoming depressed and overwrought. However, when there is obstruction of feelings and chronic bottled-up frustration, this may well result in anger alternating with depression. A depression of a liver nature invariably follows periods of long term stress and pressure which ultimately take their toll on the individual.

Addictions are closely related to the liver, be they related to alcohol, drugs or food. The emotional tension that gives rise to addictions is felt in the liver. As the liver is a powerful detoxifying plant, it becomes a dumping ground for those poisonous aspects of our being which we feel we cannot express: hatred, envy, rage, jealousy and self-disgust. If these emotions accumulate in the liver, they will weaken it and impair its function. If negative feelings and thoughts build up, this can have a detrimental affect on the immune system and the body's ability to cope with infections. The energy generated from particular repressed emotions accumulates in the form of tension and bunched muscles in our shoulders, neck and back. When the emotion is anger, the specific sentiment associated with the liver and gall bladder, backache can occur in the middle part of the back.

Coming to terms with anger and feeling OK about releasing this is an important part of getting better. Sometimes it may not be advisable to let your frustrations out in a public way. In these cases, find somewhere quiet and private, then re-enact the scenario that led to your frustration and anger. Visualize the person or situation and say exactly what you would have liked to have said earlier on, no holds barred! Alternatively, writing your feelings down on paper in the form of a letter could be helpful. You are not actually going to send it to the person concerned, so give full vent to your anger. If your emotions are severely repressed and you cannot even get in touch with your anger (another sign of an imbalance of the liver), it may be worth seeing a fully trained counsellor who can help you to get in touch with these feelings and learn to express them.

When liver *qi* starts to stagnate due to frustrations at home, work or school, an excellent way of handling them is to go to a quiet space and physically get the anger out by punching the air, a pillow or the bed, or stamping your feet and punching your fists out at the same time. Making the sound 'HO HO HO HO HO' (a technique used by certain Native American tribes; *see page 22*), in a very definite and powerful voice (not the jolly 'ho ho ho' that Santa Claus makes!), also works wonders. Once you have physically begun to release the anger held within it is ideal to follow with the wood meditation – Resolving Anger, to help pacify the soul and heal your conditions and body.

The liver is known as the body's planner or internal filofax, together with its partner organ the gall bladder, which is responsible for decision-making. If there is any stagnation in the liver, then both indecisive and disorganized behaviour will be apparent. So any problems relating to either poor planning and time management, or conversely being a fanatical filofax freak and meticulously planning everything to the last detail, can point to a liver imbalance.

On a more spiritual level, the liver is where the Hun or spiritual soul lives. The Hun hates alcohol, poisons and emotions such as anger; when these are present the Hun is said to flee from the body, which can be disastrous! However, good deeds and acts of compassion will encourage it to return! The 'Hun' or soul thrives on having a sense of purpose and vision; without these it becomes discontented and despairing, stagnation of liver *qi* contributing to this loss of aspiration and motivation. At this level, certain oils and flower remedies can be extremely beneficial in bringing harmony back to mind, body and spirit (*see pages 204–206*).

## the 9 ways to health

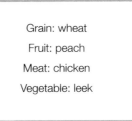

### way 1: chinese and natural nutrition

#### FOODS FOR THE WOOD ELEMENT

Grain: wheat

Fruit: peach

Meat: chicken

Vegetable: leek

#### DIETARY TIPS

1  In early Spring (the season associated with the Wood Element), eat warm foods such as stir-fries, adding more and more green vegetables that grow at this time, such as spring greens, mustard greens, romaine lettuce, radish leaves, watercress, spinach and sorrel. Include small salads in the diet again.

2  Unadulterated, unrefined, natural foods help to keep the liver healthy and efficient. A diet composed of whole grains, fresh

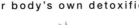

vegetables, beans, sea vegetables (nori, wakame and kombu) and fish (the diet humans are thought to have evolved on) provides optimum nutrition without any chemical toxins or excessive fats.

3   A very powerful yet simple and cheap remedy to help with liver stagnation is a drink made from 240 ml hot water and 1 tablespoon of apple vinegar. One contraindication, however, is if there are a lot of heat signs within the body. A better choice would be fresh lemon juice which is a little 'cooler' energetically than vinegar.

### Foods that strengthen the Liver and Wood Element
*(also see Recipes, page 286)*:

❋   Protect the liver and lower cholesterol by sprinkling lecithin granules over your food – this works in the same way as high-density lipoproteins (HDL), which is made up mostly of lecithin. It has a detergent action that breaks up cholesterol in the body.

❋   Dandelions are an excellent natural source of lecithin and make an interesting addition to your salad.

❋   Your liver makes about 80% of the cholesterol in your body and the consumption of saturated fats and refined sugars have been shown to increase cholesterol levels. Having oat bran porridge for breakfast can help to lower cholesterol by up to 10%.

❋   Sesame seeds can also be sprinkled over dishes and are superb for the liver as they contain protein (with eight of the important amino acids), B vitamins and vitamin E.

❋   Chicory reduces heat in the liver and benefits the gall bladder. It is particularly helpful for jaundice-type hepatitis.

❋   Strawberries tone the liver and kidneys, and are good for combating excessive urination and dizziness.

❋   Rabbit liver is good for dizziness too and sharpens the vision.

❋   Other beneficial foods for liver function are globe artichokes, asparagus, berries, buckwheat, cabbage, carrots, celery, dandelion, fennel, garlic, onion, leek, lemon, millet, oily fish, olives, parsley, parsnips, onion, brown rice, sesame oil, sunflower seeds and turmeric.

- ❋ Wholefoods such as quinoa and amaranth are particularly beneficial for the liver.
- ❋ When there is a deficiency of blood in the body this can cause an imbalance in the liver as well as the brain, other vital organs, muscles and every part of us, as blood nourishes them all. (*Please refer to the list of blood building foods on page 70.*)
- ❋ Taking essential fatty acids (*see page 16*) in the diet is highly supportive to the liver; they are best ingested on an empty stomach first thing in the morning to help flush the liver, or taken at night before bed, as the Wood Element is in power between 11 p.m. and 3 a.m.
- ❋ A useful vitamin supplement is an antioxidant formula containing selenium, vitamins C and E and beta carotene, all of which help to prevent free radical damage in the liver. One of the most comprehensive formulas available is Omnium by Solgar which is an advanced phytonutrient-rich multiple vitamin and mineral formula.
- ❋ Blue-green algae is an excellent nutrient to take to support the liver, as it not only encourages liver rejuvenation but detoxifies. Its colour is traditionally thought to reduce heat in the liver. Do ensure that the algae comes from the Upper Klamath Lake as this is the purest source, such as the certified organic Klamath Blue Green Algae or try Body Wisdom Organics Living Organics Superfood Formula which contains this Klamath Blue Green algae along with other living green super foods and special herbs to balance the five elements, including turmeric for the liver (*see page 16*).
- ❋ Kelp is a useful supplement to take if there is liver stagnation. Alternatively, include more seaweed in your diet (*see page 132*)
- ❋ Artichokes have an action on both the liver and gall bladder and can help to detoxify an overworked and congested liver. They are also helpful for anaemia as they are rich in minerals and can strengthen brittle, weak nails.

**Foods that weaken the Liver and Wood Element:**

- ❋ Foods which are **not recommended** include saturated fats (cheeses, cream, eggs and fat from meat), chocolate, coffee, oranges, pears, peanuts and nuts in general, sulphured dried fruits, chemical additives and refined convenience foods.
- ❋ As the liver plays a major role in the breakdown in the metabolism of alcohol, drinking in excess will weaken this organ. Typical hangover symptoms such as nausea, headaches, irritability, aggression, rudeness, and depression are also all signs of an imbalanced liver energy.

### Cleansing the Liver

Cleansing the liver has always been a priority in naturopathic medicine over the centuries. It is particularly beneficial for those who are sluggish, over-reactive to alcohol, intolerant to certain foods and have greeny/brown or hazel eyes (according to iridology, the practice of studying the iris of the eye to make a health diagnosis, these eye-colour types are more prone to liver and digestive disturbances). If you are troubled with unpleasant odour under your arm, this can point to your liver needing a cleanse. Avoid using anti-perspirants that contain aluminium as this will suppress your body's natural cleansing reaction. Instead, try to wash more frequently and use a natural deodorant such as Origins No Offense™ which contains essential oils and smells divine or Deokrystal by Green People. When you can no longer stand the sight or smell of fried, fatty foods, this is indeed a sign that the liver is somehow out of order. Another sign on a food front is a sudden intolerance for fruit, especially oranges, as this demonstrates that the liver has lost its ability to digest fruit acids.

Prior to working on the liver, it is highly advisable to do some work on your large intestine so that any matter that needs to be cleared in the large intestine is done so before fresh toxins are released from the liver. Liver detoxification should be undertaken gradually, as alcohol, medicines and toxins can build up over many years. The liver does not send out distress signals until a symptom or disorder has made considerable progress, so it is important to take preventative steps to support this vital organ. One of the most comprehensive antioxidants available is Omium by Solgar which is an advanced phytonutrient-rich vitamin and mineral formula. Spring time is the best season of the year to properly cleanse your body but you can make a gradual start early in the year by simply increasing your vegetable intake (preferably steamed or in soups at this time to give the body the warmth it needs), have some small salads and enjoy a juice a day, energized with the ginger to tonify your body. To further flush your body out, ensure that you drink 6 glasses of warm water (boiled water that has cooled a little) a day.

*'Harper's Liver Flush'*

Make a large fresh glass of carrot juice with ginger added to give it an extra zing and to help energetically warm the juice so that it is not too cooling on the body. Use organic wherever possible.

600 g organic carrots
1 apple
1 lemon
1 inch piece of ginger
1 tablespoon of Udo's Choice Essential Fatty Acids

Simply juice all the carrots, the apple, lemon (peel and all!), the ginger and the oil. Stir with a spoon and drink immediately. To complete the regime and ensure a balanced and complete intake of nutrients, I always take 4-6 Klamath Blue-Green Algae capsules or the Living Organics Superfood Formula by Body Wisdom Organics at the same time as this is rich in natural vitamins and minerals. In Chinese Medicine, to nourish and support the blood, half a beetroot can be added to this blend. This regime should be followed for at least two weeks, preferably in the Spring or early Summer. I will often do this throughout the year, ensuring in the colder months that I either add plenty of fresh ginger or cayenne pepper to vegetable juices to balance the cold energy of the vegetables. I feel energized and invigorated after drinking fresh juices with the addition of herbs. Warning; this can become an addictive habit (a good one!). Once you have been doing this for a few weeks and personally experience the benefits, you will not want to stop!

## way 2: herbs and spices

❋ Turmeric is the key spice for the Wood Element as it can help to decongest the liver, dissolve gallstones and strengthen digestion. However, it is not to be used for acute hepatitis or jaundice or used during pregnancy. In Indian medicine, the spice is used to help soften over tight muscles and ligaments. Students of yoga take a teaspoon a day in warm milk and it is thought to improve their flexibility. I use it to flavour and colour rice too.

❋ Silymarin or milk thistle is an amazing antioxidant herb used to treat the liver and over 200 research studies show that it can both prevent and even reverse liver damage caused by environmental toxins, drugs, alcohol and chemicals in our diet. This potent liver protector is helpful for skin conditions such as psoriasis and is an important preventative herb to take if you drink a lot of alcohol. I have also used milk thistle with great success on patients suffering with PMT, which is partly attributed to a liver imbalance according to TCM.

❋ Dandelion is used in virtually every tradition as a herb to support detoxification and is among the more nutritionally rich of medicinal herbs that is commonly recommended to help with liver and gall bladder complaints. It is known to stimulate the flow of bile that is needed for the breakdown of dietary fat, and for prevention of sluggish liver and gallstones. It is also a highly effective diuretic that has the distinct advantage over commercial preparations that tend to have the side effect of eliminating potassium from the body. Dandelion root, however, is rich in potassium, which helps compensate for the depletion of this mineral.

※ Parsley too is another diuretic herb which benefits the liver and digestive system and can be included in your diet and in fresh juice. However, do not have parsley during pregnancy.

※ Feverfew has been used since the 18th century to prevent and alleviate the symptoms of migraine. You can pick one or two leaves from the plant, infuse in boiling water and drink as a tea or purchase the individual herb (organic version is by Hambledon Herbs, UK and the standardized form is from Solgar).

※ Liquorice root has a real affinity with the liver and is able to harmonize and balance the liver *qi*. Scientific evidence has shown liver-supportive attributes that may justify the herb's use in TCM as a powerful detoxifier. High doses should be avoided if suffering from high blood pressure or purchase the deglycyrrhized form.

※ Dang gui root is another liver-friendly herb which is excellent for women as it can nourish and improve the quality of blood as it is high in vitamin B12. This herb is also very beneficial in the treatment of constipation.

※ Chamomile and peppermint herbal teas are both cooling and soothing to the liver and can help ease difficult digestion and relieve nausea.

※ St John's Wort is the Prozac of the plant world and is commonly used in the treatment of mild to moderate depression (liver stagnation in TCM) and can help to relieve seasonal affective disorder (SAD).

※ Herbal Elixir by Green People is a synergistic combination of 16 organically grown cold-pressed herbs including nettles, ginger and dandelion and is designed to help detoxify your body.

※ All the above herbs ensure the smooth flow of *qi* throughout the body and emotions and work together to help relieve liver congestion and help to release stored emotions such as irritability

your body's own detoxifier

and anger. Look for herbal tincture blends (ideally organic) that include a combination of the above herbs such as the Wood Element Organic Herbal Elixir and tea blend produced by Body Wisdom Organics or purchase a standardized herb individually from a reputable company such as Solgar (available in the UK and the US).

## way 3: exercise

We need to nurture the body and prepare it for Spring as the energy begins to rise in the body after lying dormant during the Winter months. Getting involved in gentle exercise and building your programme up over the Spring is an excellent idea; a heavy exercise regime is not recommended in the early stages of Spring. The body needs time to adapt to the new season and to allow its energy to rise up gradually from within.

Some aerobic exercise and gentle stretching to increase the oxygen intake into the muscles will be supportive when liver energy is blocked. If there is extreme stagnation and inner anger, it might be worth trying kickboxing or investing in a punch bag to get those frustrations out of your body. Balance is the key here, as too much exercise and physical exertion is not good for any of the organs.

As a liver imbalance can generate stiffness in the body, stretching can soften the muscles and relieve built-up pressure. And just as liver congestion can cause the body to become inflexible and rigid, so stretching and softening your muscles will have a beneficial effect on your liver.

A specific exercise which stretches the liver and gall bladder meridian is described on *page 178*.

## way 4: massage and reflex points

The primary neuro-lymphatic point for the liver is situated on your right hand side, starting in line with your right nipple, 2-3 cm below in a curve under the breast (for ladies, this is where your bra wire lies) and across to your sternum (breast bone). This band is best massaged on a daily basis, preferably several times throughout the day as the liver needs as much support as possible with the abuse it receives in these modern times!

The liver reflex point is situated on the right foot. Gently massage the reflex using talc as a medium and finish by massaging your feet with a base oil (olive, sunflower, apricot, almond, etc.) to which has been added a few drops of your chosen essential oil. One or two suitable flower remedies (*see page 206*) can also be included in this mixture. For the best results, massage this into the acupressure point known as Liver 3 (*see page 203*) as well as the reflex point on the feet. As the liver rules the eyes, it would be a good idea to gently massage the eye reflex shown below too, if you have weak eye sight or as a preventative technique (*see below* for points). Breathe deeply, visualizing the colour green and saying the liver sound 'SHHHHHH'. Shut out all distractions, retaining your mental tranquillity. This massage and relaxation programme will provide one of the best protective remedies for the liver. (*See page 23 for massage techniques.*)

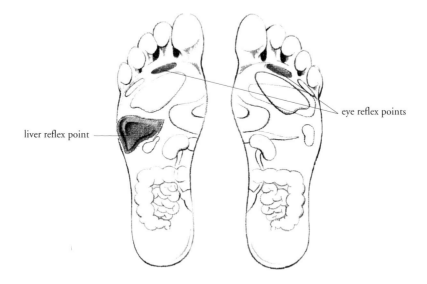

liver reflex point

eye reflex points

*Reflexology Point for the Liver (shaded)*

your body's own detoxifier

## way 5: acupressure

The liver meridian starts on the top surface of the big toe and runs up the foot, along the inside leg, around the genitals and through the liver and gall bladder. The internal pathway of the liver meridian travels from here, up the throat until it reaches the eye (this part is not shown on the diagram).

To trace the meridian, place your palms or fingers just on the inside of your big toes and run them up the inside of your legs, dropping down and looping around your genitals and out at your hips, finishing up at your ribs, just below the breast (*see diagram below*).

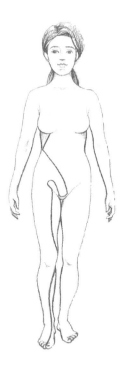

*The Liver Meridian*

*Liver 3*

This is considered to be the most important point on the liver meridian. It is located in the hollow area at the top of the foot between the first and second toes, about 2.5 cm away from the webbed part. Working this point calms the nervous system, reduces irritability and depression, strengthens the immune system and liver, prevents/relieves headaches, eases food cravings (reduces allergic sensitivity), overcomes the effects of too much exercise, stress, strains or toxins in the body and increases circulation in the legs. Using your thumb, gently rub the point, moving forwards and backwards over the area for approximately 1 to 2 minutes.

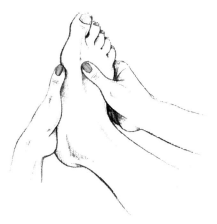

*Liver 3 Acupressure Point (under the right thumb)*

*Governor vessel 20*

This point, right on the crown of the head, is called 'the point of a thousand meetings'; it is valuable for helping to raise and disperse liver *qi*.

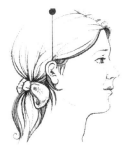

*Governor Vessel 20 Acupressure Point (draw an imaginary line from the top of the ear to the crown)*

## way 6: essential oils

**Bergamot:** harmonizes the liver *qi*, thus allowing an even flow of energy around the body. Regulates and calms the nervous system (nervous tension often being created by stagnation of *qi* in the liver). Helps to release pent-up feelings often experienced prior to a period, PMS being a classic example of stagnant liver energy. *Strength factor: Medium*

**Bitter orange:** unblocks stagnant *qi* when it builds in the liver, stomach and intestines, thereby easing emotional tension, difficulty sleeping/ insomnia and nauseous headaches or migraines. Ideal for digestive symptoms such as abdominal distension, flatulence, indigestion, nausea, vomiting and constipation. Stimulates the liver and the gall bladder, encouraging the flow of bile and thus supporting the body with the breakdown of fats. Can be useful for workaholic types who are intolerant of mistakes. Works well with the Bach Flower Remedy Rock Water (*see page 206*). Tangerine also regulates *qi* and helps alleviate nausea. *Strength factor: Medium*

**Chamomile:** eases emotional tension, frustration and depression. If the *qi* is very stuck, it can affect the flow of blood, leading to a condition known as 'blood stagnation' in Chinese medicine. This can create menstrual disorders and pain, but Chamomile's superb analgesic properties can help to reduce this pain. *Strength factor: Strong*

**Grapefruit:** cools an over-heated and abused liver. Detoxifies and cleanses the body; boosts a sluggish lymphatic system. Has a wonderful fruity, uplifting smell that can ease frustration and tension. For those with eating disorders or those who raid the refrigerator when under pressure, this oil erases the guilt, self-blame, remorse and depression that follows a 'binge'. Heals that vulnerable inner part of ourselves that was crying out for help in the first place. *Strength factor: Medium*

**Lavender:** clears anger from the liver and cleanses and soothes the spirit of anger and exhaustion. Has nerve-relaxant properties, making it ideal for releasing liver stagnation, which upsets the flow of body energy and blood and gives rise to frustration, mood swings, anger, abdominal distension, headaches and menstrual disorders. Just as it can soothe the discomfort of sunburn, lavender can also disperse some of the latent heat that can build up in the liver and generate further stagnation, as well as diffuse over-heated emotions. *Strength factor: Weak*

**Neroli:** calms the mind, relaxes the nervous system, gently lifts the spirit. Particularly comforting to 'sensitive souls' who have the tendency to over-work and drive themselves too hard, falling prey to mental and emotional exhaustion. Comforts and strengthens the mind, body and spirit, bringing them back to a point of balance and harmony. *Strength factor: Medium*

A good blended range is Origins Gloomaway™ which contains essential oils such as grapefruit, orange and mint or Body Wisdom Organics Wood Element Essential Oil Blend that includes bergamot, mandarin, lavender and grapefruit. Another excellent product is Neem Oil which is made by the Organic Herbal Cosmetic Company Dr Hauschka which is designed specifically to strengthen weak nails … and it works!

your body's own detoxifier

## way 7: flower remedies

**Impatiens:** for mood swings, impatience, anger, inner tension, a 'blowing hot and cold' disposition, over-reactions and general irritability. Eases these 'pressure cooker' feelings and generates empathy, compassion, gentleness and understanding for others.

**Rock Water:** for perfectionist individuals who constantly drive and strive and thus become over-tense and irritable. These types can be so strict and inflexible they deny themselves any pleasures, thus creating even more liver *qi* stagnation. This is a good remedy to add to your bath water (about 6 drops, possibly along with Bitter orange essential oil, which complements Rock Water well).

**Vervain:** for workaholic type personalities prone to overexertion who set up stress patterns in the body typical of liver symptoms (including headaches, physical tension, muscle congestion, migraines and eyestrain). Allows us to become more tolerant of situations, to let go and go with the flow. Channels our natural enthusiasms and leads to an altogether more calm, relaxed life.

**Dandelion:** FF12 (detox formula) dandelion, a yellow flower that stimulates the liver and supports hepatic function, can help to ease anger and temper tantrums by lessening the impact of aggression and promotes a caring, cherishing and calm attitude.

Alternatively, try the Phytobiophysics Liver Meridian Formula or the Wood Element Flower Formula by Body Wisdom Organics which contains the liver and gall bladder meridian formulas in an organic herbal flower base.

You may also find some appropriate flower remedies for supporting the Wood Element in the chapter on the gall bladder (*page 000*).

## way 8: affirmations

- ❋ I respect and entrust my liver to perform its many varied and complex functions.
- ❋ I feel calm, confident and able to organize and plan my life.
- ❋ I am flexible and yielding, my body moves with grace and ease.
- ❋ The life force (or *qi*) moves freely throughout my mind and body, dispersing any congestion.
- ❋ I fill my liver with a healing green light which calms my spirit, dissolves tension and fills me with a sense of peace and wellbeing.

*See also the Gall Bladder chapter, page 184, for affirmations that may be used in conjunction with these.*

07

## way 9: meditation for soul nourishment

*See Gall Bladder chapter, page 184.*

# understanding the metal element

The key to

- ✳ Boosting your Immune System
- ✳ Better Breathing
- ✳ Super Skin
- ✳ Letting Go of Grief
- ✳ Eliminating Toxins from your Bowels

**Partner Organs:** The lungs and large intestine are the partner organs for the Metal Element. The lungs expel carbon dioxide, and the large intestine eliminates solid residue. If this waste is not eliminated frequently it can have an effect on the skin. The skin is known in TCM as 'the third lung'; it is part of the Metal Element and can reflect sluggish bowels (toxins that remain in the colon for too long will be discharged through the skin). The bowel is one of the most important routes of elimination for self-cleansing, and works together with the kidneys, bladder, lungs and skin to help eliminate waste efficiently from the body. It contains friendly bacteria which can synthesize B vitamins and help to keep the level of harmful, pathogenic bacteria to a minimum.

**Climate:** Dryness: a passion for dry weather or, conversely, a hatred of it point to a Metal Element imbalance. In nature, Autumn reflects dryness, as seen in the leaves when they lose their moisture, shrivel up and 'let go' of the branches they have hung on to since Springtime.

**Season:** Autumn, the time to reflect on the past year and to prepare for withdrawing as the Winter months close in. It is a time to protect the back of the neck from the winds, which begin to get cooler, otherwise you will be more susceptible to minor illnesses after the hot Summer months.

**Colour:** White. Someone obsessed with wearing white or who strongly dislikes the colour can be demonstrating an imbalance in the Metal Element. A white hue coming off the face is also indicative of lung problems according to TCM, just as a very white or pale skin in Western medicine is considered a sign that the lungs are too tight or there is local congestion, constricting the circulation.

**Time of day:** 3–5 a.m. (lungs): if there are problems with this organ you may wake up between these times and even experience breathing difficulties. This shows that there are unresolved issues around the emotion of grief, which corresponds to the Metal Element. Extreme grief is injurious to the lungs, and a person who is going through a period of grieving will often have bowel problems. The time of day for the large intestine is 5–7 a.m.; according to TCM this is the best time of day to have your first bowel movement. If there are any imbalances in the bowel, getting up between these times will encourage the body to rid itself efficiently of toxins held in the bowel.

**Body Tissue:** The skin is seen as the third lung and breathes just as surely and necessarily as the lungs themselves. The link between lung problems and the skin is quite well documented in Western medicine: it is common for children who have been given suppressive skin treatments for eczema to go on to develop asthma. It is known that many skin problems such as psoriasis, eczema, rough, dry skin and rashes reflect an imbalance in the body that relates directly to the lungs. The correlation of the skin with the lungs and respiratory function is an important diagnostic tool in Chinese medicine. Elimination is also associated with the skin, since the skin is involved in the process of ridding the body of wastes. In Japan there is also an ancient belief that the skin reflects the condition of the internal organs: if the latter are fatigued in any way, it will reflect on our skin. Dead sea salts can greatly improve the texture and appearance of your skin. They are an extremely rich source of minerals including potassium, magnesium and calcium. These relaxing and restorative minerals allow for the absorption of more moisture, contributing to softer, smoother skin. Good products that I have tried include Aveda's Soothing Aqua Therapy™ which is combined with plant-based emollients and essences to rehydrate and heal your skin. Origins have several products with dead sea salts including Go for the Glow™ mineral salt body scrub. Remember too with dry and flaky skin, there is often a deficiency in essential fatty acids so ensure that you eat plenty of oily fish and seeds and supplement with an oil rich in omega 3 and 6 essential fatty acids such as Udo's Choice oil.

**Voice sound:** The sound of the Metal Element is a weeping tone of voice, which does not always coincide with actual tears. There is often a sense of sadness and loss, grief being the emotion of the Metal Element. The voice will invariably be very soft, too, almost angelic or ethereal.

**Sense Organ:** We usually breathe through the nose. In TCM, the lungs are never separated from the nose, which is the sense organ of the Metal Element. Problems which affect the nose have a direct bearing on the lungs; equally, lung problems are often accompanied by disturbances in the nasal fluids. The secretion for this element is mucus, from any of the mucous membranes in the body. A deficiency of mucus can show that the body is over-heated, causing dryness on the surface of the skin. Alternatively, an excessive amount of mucus indicates an imbalance in the lungs. Therefore, dryness in the throat or nose, coughing, difficulty breathing, aching in the lungs, rasping, nasal drip and sinus blockages can all be related to the Metal Element is not properly balanced.

**Reflector:** Body hair is the physical manifestation of the Metal Element. Excessive body hair or the loss of body hair points to an imbalance. The hair on our head, however, is ruled by the kidneys.

**Symptoms of Imbalance:** Oedema, wet skin, excessive mucus and abnormal perspiration patterns are connected with the lungs, as the lungs, along with the Water Element, play an important role in the regulation of body fluids. Conversely, deficiencies of moisture can cause severe dryness in the body, signs of which may be lack of secretions, emaciation, anaemia, poor appetite and a white, ethereal appearance. The skin will be tight and therefore perspiration sparse. The large intestine has the ability, on a higher level, to generate movement forwards in our lives, encouraging evolution and change. Constriction and cynical behaviour patterns emerge if the energy of the large intestine is poor. In TCM, nose bleeds, sore throat, neck swelling, thirst and a dry mouth, toothache and pain along the relevant meridian are all symptoms of an imbalance in the large intestine. When there are intestinal disorders, including chronic constipation, the blood can become congested in the colon.

# your body's own ventilator

\* \* \* \* \* \* \* \* \* \* \* \* \* \* \* \* \* \* \* \* \* \* \* \* \* \*

## what your lungs do for you

We all know the relaxing and soothing feeling of breathing deeply and slowly. The calming effect of drawing oxygen into the lungs is an amazing process. Our lungs truly give the body the wonderful breath of life. The lungs are very sensitive and can be damaged in various ways from pollutants in our environment to the emotional stress in our life. Physical symptoms can surface such as shortness of breath, nasal difficulties, eczema and more chronic conditions like asthma or emphysema. In TCM, emotional symptoms such as grief, apathy, melancholy and pessimism can also appear as a direct result of lung disorders.

### TRADITIONAL WESTERN UNDERSTANDING

The main function of the lungs is to supply the body with oxygen, which is transported through the circulatory system in the blood. The 'used' air, which is composed of toxins and carbon dioxide, is released by the lungs when we exhale.

Good lung ventilation is assured by clean air and healthy lung tissue. Sadly, with our environmental conditions worsening year by year, the functioning of our lungs is often impaired. Every part of our body, from our organs to our blood and cells, can be poisoned by what is absorbed from the external environment. Our internal environment can also have a great impact on our lungs. Emotional stresses can result in constriction of the lungs, thus preventing an efficient changeover of nutrients in the blood.

Weakness in the lungs manifest in susceptibility to asthma, emphysema, bronchitis and infections of the throat, sinuses and chest. Air pollution and high stress levels can weaken the immune system and lungs and contribute to allergic reactions such as hayfever and asthma. Having very white or pale skin can indicate a deficiency of haemoglobin (the protein that carries oxygen and iron) in the blood and possibly lung weakness. Smoking injures the lungs and creates heat and dryness; excessive consumption of fat also weakens the lungs as too much cholesterol and fat in the bloodstream reduce the oxygen-carrying capacity of the blood. The dangers of smoking are well documented, but one interesting fact that is not so widely known is that smokers mix tiny amounts of nicotine into their saliva. This then has an impact on digestion as it inhibits the production of gastric juices in the stomach.

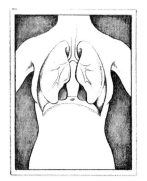

The lungs are cone-shaped organs located inside the rib cage and separated from the abdominal organs by a sheet of muscle called the diaphragm.

## TRADITIONAL CHINESE INTERPRETATION

| | |
|---|---|
| Element: | Metal |
| Partner organ: | Large intestine |
| Climate: | Dryness |
| Season: | Autumn |
| Colour: | White |
| Time of day: | 3–5 a.m. |
| Body tissue: | Skin |
| Voice sound: | Weeping |
| Sense organ: | Nose |
| Reflector: | Body Hair |
| Taste: | Spicy |
| Emotion: | Grief |

## SYMPTOMS OF IMBALANCE

### Physical Symptoms

Breathing difficulties • Asthma, emphysema
• Shortness of breath • Very soft voice • Coughing,
throat problems • Sinusitis • Psoriasis, eczema, dry skin
• Nasal difficulties • Excessive or lack of perspiration •
Mucus or dryness in the body • Poor sense of smell •
Aversion to dryness

In Traditional Chinese Medicine it is believed that the lungs extract clean *qi* from the inhaled air and combine this with food *qi* from the spleen. The lungs spread *qi* all over the body to nourish the tissues and promote

*your body's own ventilator*

all physiological processes. The lungs govern the breath and are responsible for the production of 'defensive *qi*'. This *qi* is said to protect us from damaging external climatic factors such as wind, cold and damp, to which the lungs are quite vulnerable. The lungs disperse this 'defensive *qi*' to fluids found in the spaces between the skin and muscles throughout the body. This function ensures defensive *qi* is equally distributed under the skin and can perform its role in warming the skin and muscles, so protecting the body. If the lung energy is weak, our resistance will be lowered and we will be more prone to infections.

The respiratory function affects all the rhythms of the body/mind, including blood flow. Breathing, along with food, is one of the main ways to replenish the body and its energy levels. However, because it is so simple and basic to life, breathing often can be overlooked until a specific problem arises such as asthma or shortness of breath.

The highest function of the lungs, according to the Chinese, is that they act as the Receiver of Energy, taking energy from the outside into ourselves, on every level. We breathe emotionally as well as physically – the expressions *breathless with excitement* and *breathtaking* give us a hint of this. The larynx is part of the respiratory system, so the lung meridian controls the voice. When your tone of voice is quiet, this can indicate that the state of *qi* within the body is quite deficient.

### Emotional Symptoms

Grief • Being unable to let go • Apathy, boredom • Lack of inspiration • Melancholy • Pessimism • Remote, distant behaviour

Traditional Chinese Medicine associates prolonged sorrow and grief with the lungs. Grief is a natural, human emotion like all the emotions we experience, but someone who is constantly overwhelmed by sorrow is considered to be suffering an imbalance afflicting the organs of the Metal Element.

The lungs are very much involved with the process of 'letting go'. After all, if the lungs did not 'let go' of the carbon dioxide and other toxins that are expelled during expiration, then we would be in trouble! The letting go of emotions, grief and sadness has just as much relevance: if these emotions are held inside over time, then we put ourselves at risk of developing physical ailments.

The lungs receive what is termed as 'heavenly *qi*', thought to provide inspiration and a sense of meaning in life. If the energy flow is poor, apathy, boredom and a lack of inspiration and meaning in life may be the result. The Bodily Soul, or P'o as it is called by the Chinese, is believed to live in the lungs and is easily affected by negative emotions, especially those of remorse and pessimism. If one has never truly grieved over a loss, it can develop into a Metal Element depression which manifests as an inability to progress in life.

# the 9 ways to health

## way 1: chinese and natural nutrition

### FOODS FOR THE METAL ELEMENT

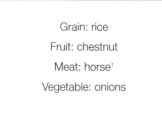

Grain: rice
Fruit: chestnut
Meat: horse[1]
Vegetable: onions

If an element is out of balance, the right foods help restore it. A combination of foods for all the elements is a healthy, balanced diet.

### DIETARY TIPS

1   As one of the symptoms of imbalance for the lungs is lack of inspiration, try and be creative with your cooking! Motivate yourself to combine different textures, colours and flavours in your meals so that it becomes an exciting, new visual treat!
2   Conquer apathy and boredom through having a different perspective and attitude towards eating. Be inventive in the kitchen and seek out healthy alternatives and keep remembering that this is an opportunity to let go of old habits and nourish the new!

---

[1] While horse meat is recommended for this element, I do not condone its consumption.

### Foods that strengthen the Lungs and Metal Element

*(also see Recipes, page 288)*:

- The flavour associated with the Metal Element is pungent and spicy, referring to curries, spices and peppery foods. Excess pungent foods make the muscles knotty and the finger and toe nails weak, according to ancient Chinese texts. The pungency goes directly to the respiratory tract, so it is important to moderate your intake of these foods. However, other organs can benefit from this flavour: if, for example, the kidneys suffer from dryness, pungent foods will moisten them.

- Common foods in Chinese Medicine to enhance lung function are carrots, button mushrooms, crab apples, olives, pears, radishes, tangerines, walnuts, water chestnuts and wine.

- Peaches and green onions are known to stop perspiration.

- Hot peppers (the active compound being capsaicin) have been used for centuries in Traditional Chinese Medicine for any type of respiratory problem. Today, peppers are recommended to strengthen the respiratory system and so are valuable to include in your diet if you are (or have been) a smoker or if you are suffering from congestion from a cold or sinus disorder.

- In natural medicine, onions, garlic, scallions, chives and leeks (all part of the allium group) have been used to treat chest complaints and help keep the airways open and clear. Garlic could be considered as an agent to strengthen our defensive *qi*, which helps us to fight infections as it possesses compounds that help to destroy infection-causing bacteria and can help to boost our immune system.

- The effects of smoking can stay in the body for many years, so even if you no longer currently smoke, it is important to make sure that your diet is high in anti-oxidants. These nutrients can help prevent the damage to the lungs associated with smoking. Good food sources include yellow/orange coloured vegetables and green leafy vegetables.

- Other supportive foods are watercress, mustard and cress, turnips, Chinese cabbage and celery. Apples, apricots, egg whites, mandarins, strawberries and peanuts all help to lubricate the lungs.

**your body's own ventilator**

**Foods that weaken the Lungs and Metal Element:**

❋ Dairy products (especially taken cold) and orange juice should be avoided if there is any sign of mucus in the body, as they can increase mucus production.

## way 2: herbs and spices

❋ Thyme is the key spice or culinary herb that I have chosen for the Metal Element. It is often used in teas to help ease conditions such as bronchitis and other respiratory complaints due to its potent bactericidal properties. The tea can also be used as a gargle to soothe sore throats and coughs.

❋ Astragalus is a very popular tonic herb in Chinese medicine that can help to strengthen and build resistance to infection. It has been shown to shorten the duration of the common cold and protect against numerous other viruses.

❋ Echinacea has active compounds that can help to reinforce the body's own defence mechanism and is well known for its ability to accelerate recovery from infections, colds and flu by enhancing our immunity. Trials have shown that this herb is more potent when taken intensively in the early stages of infection and over a two week period without interruption, in a similar fashion to an antibiotic.

❋ Elacampane is used for coughs, excess mucus and is seen in herbalism as being particularly helpful for conditions such as bronchitis and asthma.

❋ Hyssop is another herb used for chronic mucus, as well as used for coughs and bronchitis.

❋ Hippocrates and Dioscorides both used coltsfoot for all lung and chest disorders. It is an excellent herb that can help to loosen mucus, give relief to a hoarse throat and other respiratory conditions.

❋ Ginger too is used for any conditions where the body is not coping effectively with balancing its moisture level as it can help to dry up excess mucus.

❋ Spicy teas such as Hambledon Herbs organic Spice Delight or Yogi tea contain spices such as cinnamon, clove, cardamom, black pepper and ginger which can be very warming to take if you are coming down with a cold or flu.

❋ Garlic has an affinity with the lung: if you rub your feet with a clove of garlic, in 15 minutes your breath will smell of it! It can also help to reduce the amount of mucus produced by the body.

❋ Look for herbal tincture blends or teas that include some of the above herbs such as the Metal Element Organic Herbal Elixir and tea produced by Body Wisdom Organics. If you are looking for individual supplements, Solgar's range of herbs includes astragalus, garlic, echinacea and ginger.

## way 3: exercise

Vigorous cardiovascular exercise obviously has a beneficial effect on the lungs as breathing becomes more frequent and deeper. Too much lying down can damage the lung and large intestine meridians, affecting both elimination and respiration. To remedy this, work on acupressure point Large Intestine 4, located in the muscle between the thumb and first finger, and on Large Intestine 11, found at the elbow crease on the outer part of the arm (*see diagram, page 248*).

The stretch for the lung and large intestine meridians involves clasping your hands behind your back and bending forward gently, keeping your knees unlocked. Lift your arms as high as possible behind you. Hold and breathe deeply. Repeat three times then relax; follow with some deep breathing exercises. Remember that it may take weeks or months to achieve this. Work at your own pace and ensure that you have warmed the muscles in your body for 10 minutes prior to stretching. If possible, join a local yoga class where you can be guided and personally instructed.

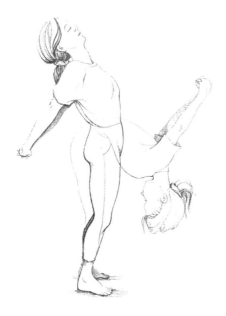

*The Lung/Large Intestine Stretch*

**Breathing Exercises**

Breathing exercises are an essential part of any self-healing programme. The rise and the fall of the lungs and diaphragm will directly affect the internal organs positively, as the movement massages them internally. Practising this on a daily basis, along with following the other guidelines recommended in this book, will keep the internal organs in top form.

Deep breathing gives us the breath of life and puts us in touch with ourselves. It is believed to be the interface between body and mind. Learning how to breathe deeply and fully can help us to experience a new awakening of energy and a greater enthusiasm for life. Conversely, shallow breathing or breathing difficulties can cause the body to become sluggish and toxic, hampering the healing process. It is essential that the organs, tissues and cells all receive an adequate supply of oxygen to allow them to carry out their duties efficiently.

**Breath of Life Exercise**

Lying or sitting in a comfortable position, place one hand on your lower abdomen and one on your chest. Take a slow, deep breath, allowing the air to flow down to your abdomen. Feel your lower hand rise as the air fills this area. At the same time, notice whether there is much movement of the hand that is on your chest. The ultimate aim is that the hand on your abdomen should rise and fall with your breathing, while the hand on your chest remains relatively still. Exhale slowly, allowing your abdomen and lungs to deflate properly. Again, focus on your lower hand rising as you inhale fresh, clean air. Hold the breath for a few seconds and, on exhaling, allow your abdomen to collapse, ensuring that all the stale air that you have been storing in your body is released. Do this three times and then relax into a natural pattern of breathing.

If there is grieving or sadness, back pain will be felt between the shoulder blades. Massaging the sternum can also help, using small circular movements, noting any sensitive spots and gently working on them (*see Heart chapter, page 99*).

## way 4: massage and reflex points

To stimulate the neuro-lymphatic points for your lungs, massage your sternum starting at the top and work down in small spirals until you reach the tip of your sternum. Points are also located on either side of the sternum (*see page 225*), so massage here too and spend time on any congested or sore areas. Another very powerful point to energize the immune system is located approximately 4-5 cm beneath your collar bone on the sternum. Tapping it (and some even recommend thumping it like a gorilla does in the jungle!) for about 30 seconds will help to re-align and stimulate your energy. It is even more powerful when combined with two other significant neuro-lymphatic points – the kidney (*page 160*) and the spleen (*page 75*).

The ball of the foot is the area that connects to the lungs; as we have both a right and a left lung, the points are found on both feet. Holding your left foot, massage the ball of the foot, noting any sore areas or gritty parts. These 'crystals' are a build-up of uric acid that can quite easily break down. However, don't endeavour to get rid of them all in one or two sessions. Try and massage your foot every day or every other day, just for a couple of minutes. *(See page 23 for massage techniques.)*

To help clear any sinus congestion, gently massage the pads of the toes.

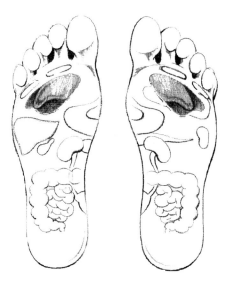

*Reflexology Points for the Lungs (shaded)*

When doing any of the above exercises, always make the lung sound 'SSSSSSS' as you exhale, slowly controlling your breath and visualizing a white, healing light flowing in during inhalation. See it entering your lungs and permeating the oxygen molecules so that this white light is carried all around the body, thus promoting healing on a very deep level.

## way 5: acupressure

The meridian for the lungs has an internal branch which begins near the stomach and goes upwards through the upper body cavity, surfacing below the clavicle (Lung 1). It then runs down the lateral side of the left arm and finishes on the outside of the thumb nail. Take one hand to lung 1 and take your palm up towards your shoulder and down the inside of your arm, finishing by sweeping off your thumb. Repeat on the other side.

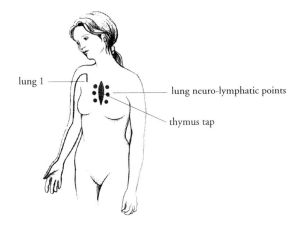

*The Lung Meridian*

Acupressure has been found to be extremely beneficial for most lung imbalances. A study of asthma patients in the US revealed that their lung capacity increased after a 20-minute acupressure session.

### Lung 1

This point is found on the outer part of the chest, about 2.5–5 cm beneath the collarbone. It is one of the main points to help release tension caused by emotional stress. Holding it relieves difficult breathing and asthma symptoms, and releases suppressed grief.

## Lung 7

This point greatly strengthens the lungs and entire respiratory system. It is located 2.5 cm from the wrist crease on the inside of the forearm, in line with the thumb. It is a good preventative point for breathing difficulties and congestion, and also helps to relieve coughs and colds, especially in the early stages. It can help to revitalize and lift the spirits, as it helps to move and circulate lung *qi*. It is also a useful point for easing a runny nose and correcting a loss of the sense of smell.

226

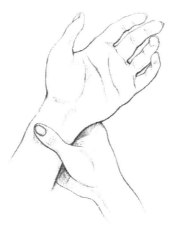

*Lung 7 Acupressure Point (under the thumb)*

## way 6: essential oils

**Clary Sage:** strengthens lung energy and soothes a constricted chest. Restores our inner reserves when they are weak and vulnerable. Contains the plant hormones known as phyto-oestrogens, so use with care. *Strength factor: Strong*

nine ways to body wisdom

**Cypress:** strengthens and supports the Bodily Soul and heavenly *qi*. Relaxes breathing and encourages us to flow on an emotional level, taking in the new and releasing the old. Helps in times of change and upheaval. *Strength factor: Medium*

**Eucalyptus:** a classic respiratory oil which has a very strong connection to the lung area. Anticatarrhal, antibacterial and anti-viral; unmatched for its powerful action on lung infections, sinusitis and even the common cold. Clears mucus and decongests lungs and whole body, supporting and enhancing immune system functioning. Lifts the spirits, dispersing any negative feelings of suffocation or grief. *Strength factor: Strong*

**Frankincense:** strengthens the defensive *qi* and so greatly supports and protects the immune system. Calming, helping to deepen the breath and slow down respiration. Ideal for asthma, as it can help to relieve tightness in the chest, and for conditions such as bronchitis. Possesses expectorant and anti-catarrhal properties. *Strength factor: Strong*

**Pine:** like eucalyptus is a powerful antiseptic oil that is used for breathlessness and can help your body to fight colds and lung infections. Has a beneficial effect on the skin and is used for eczema and psoriasis. Pine is revered as a herb of protection and so can help to strengthen our spiritual defences when our *qi* is low and we are more susceptible to negative energy. *Strength factor: Medium*

**Tea Tree:** possesses supreme antifungal and antiviral properties together with being a powerful natural antibiotic. Strengthens weak lung *qi*, thus easing symptoms such as shallow breathing, chronic weakness, mental fatigue and general immune disorders. Increases our resistance to disease so is a perfect choice for vulnerable, weak, susceptible individuals who are prone to catching common infections. Can help to boost morale after a debilitating illness. *Strength factor: Strong*

**Thyme:** an extremely 'hot' anti-infectious oil that has a very invigorating effect on both the physical and mental plane. Uplifts, tones and strengthens weak lung energy; can help to ease conditions such as chronic fatigue syndrome, white or clear catarrh and coughs, and opens the chest thus helping improve shallow breathing. Lifts us out of melancholy and grief by enhancing the heavenly *qi*. *Strength factor: Strong*

It is always best to seek advice from a trained aromatherapist or herbalist who can assess your individual needs. For example, with a condition such as asthma, the choice of oils could depend on whether the asthma was emotionally based or caused by an allergy or infection.

Other oils of benefit include **Rose**, **Lavender**, **Neroli**, **Chamomile** and **Bergamot** (for their anti-spasmodic, anti-inflammatory and anti-depressant properties), along with **Sandalwood**, **Marjoram**, **Myrrh** and **Benzoin**.

Good blends include Nothing to Sneeze At™ by Origins which contains Laurel and Eucalyptus, or Body Wisdom Organics Metal Element Organic Essential Oil Blend which contains pine, tea tree, thyme and eucalyptus.

## way 7: flower remedies

**Honeysuckle:** for those who just cannot seem to move on; a good remedy for grief as it helps to dissolve remorse and regrets about the past. Makes us feel more focused and aware of the present. Can also be used for childhood traumas that haunt you, and in times of bereavement where it is extremely difficult to get over the loss of a loved one.

**Hornbeam:** the remedy for that 'Monday morning feeling', when you feel lethargic, weary, apathetic, unmotivated and bored. Helps to encourage us to face the day with renewed vigour and a freshness of mind and body. Revitalizes and strengthens the heavenly *qi*, thus providing more meaning and inspiration in your life.

**Pine:** has a highly therapeutic action on the lungs. Recommended for people who blame themselves and carry guilt, feeling responsible for the actions of others. Helps to dissolve guilt and remorse and enables us to distinguish when a problem is ours and when it is someone else's.

**Water Violet:** for those who withdraw into their own little world for protection. They cannot let people into their space or 'receive' the richness of human experience and advice. Helps to break down the walls that surround them, allowing others to come closer and yet still retain their serenity and poise.

**Wild Rose:** for dullness and fatigue when the energy flow of heavenly *qi* is low and there is no sense of meaning in life. Revives the spirit and renews our sense of joy, bringing new levels of inspiration and motivation.

**Nicotiana:** FF10 or the Breath of Life flower formula can help to support the immune system. Emotionally it improves self worth and promotes a forgiving nature, so enabling us to release hurt and rejection.

**Phacelia:** FF6 is another formula for the immune system which can help with sinus problems and excess mucus.

**Nightshade:** FF5 or Imu-Ace is designed to help strengthen the immune system.

**Lotus Vitality:** FF1 balances the Govenor vessel and is also used as an amplifier for the lung meridian.

Alternatively, try the Phytobiophysics Lung Meridian Formula or the Metal Element Flower Formula by Body Wisdom Organics which contains the large intestine and lung meridian formulas in an organic herbal flower base.

You may also find some appropriate flower remedies for supporting the Metal Element in the Large Intestine chapter (*page 249*).

## way 8: affirmations

- ❋ I now expand my lungs and breathe deeply, so inhaling the sustaining breath of life.
- ❋ With every breath I take, I feel protected and uplifted by the life force.
- ❋ I now let go of any sadness and pain that I have experienced in my past.
- ❋ I am filled with inspiration and divine energy.

See also the Large Intestine chapter, *page 250*, for affirmations that may be used in conjunction with these.

## way 9: meditation for soul nourishment ... releasing grief and letting go

Before beginning this meditation exercise, familiarize yourself with the diagrams of the relevant meridians (i.e. for the lungs and large intestine).

Visualize yourself sitting beneath the boughs of a mighty oak tree in Autumn. Notice the leaves on the different trees in the wood and see the rich variations in colour from red to russet and gold set against the early evening sky. This time of year represents the drawing in and bringing to a close the earlier seasons of growth and abundance. Just as nature has to let go of her fruits and leaves, so we can begin to let go of ideas and thoughts that no longer have relevance in our life. Focus more closely on a branch of a tree with its leaves about to fall. As you watch, a yellow leaf falls gently to the earth. Imagine that this falling leaf represents a feeling, an event or a relationship that you need to let go of. Do not be scared of experiencing loss – try and understand that loss is a necessary part of our life's cycle. Give yourself permission to feel any sorrow or grief as you release the memory. Continue this process of attaching emotions or events to various leaves on the branch until you feel that you have let go of negative thoughts and feelings which are no longer necessary in your life. Follow each leaf as it falls from the tree on the ground and give thanks that you have been able to let go of these attachments. View the pile of leaves that have been released from the tree lying on the ground. Allow time to speed up and see the leaves decomposing and rotting into the earth, providing nourishment for new growth. For the cycle of life, it is necessary to release what is no longer needed, to allow for the process of re-birth and regeneration to begin. See little tiny green shoots appearing where the leaves once lay reflecting new openings and new beginnings. Fill your body with light and hope of a brighter future where new doors will open and take you on rich, life-enhancing journeys where you will experience many fascinating and wonderful things.

Now visualize a beautiful white light entering the top of your head. Feel this healing white light as it gently cleanses your mind, and know deep within that by releasing the old, you have created room for new, fresh and positive thoughts and feelings. Feel the sense of peace, clarity and calmness that this realization brings. In your own time, allow the white light to flow down into your neck and shoulders, releasing any stiffness held in this area of your body. Notice if you are carrying a heavy burden – do you still need to carry this and is it really yours to carry? Mentally picture this as a back pack that has been pulling heavily on your shoulders and back. Ease the straps and slip it off your shoulders. Set it down and view the contents. Is it really necessary to be carrying all of those things around with you every moment of the day? Probably not, so leave the bag on the ground and focus on your shoulders – feel the sense of relief and release as you no longer carry those burdens on your back. Now concentrate and intensify the white light and allow it to flow to your chest and into your lungs. Allow your breath to deepen – inhale the clear white light and exhale any remaining stresses and strains that are still being processed.

your body's own ventilator

Now visualize the *qi* flowing towards the lung meridian beginning on the front of your shoulder. Build the *qi* here at the acupressure point lung 1 and allow it to help dissolve any further grief that you may be feeling emotionally or physically. Allow this grief and sorrow to leave your body through your exhalation and allow the new air on your in-breath to heal and cleanse. Send the white light down the meridian along the outside of your arm until it reaches the inside of your thumb. Next, allow the *qi* to flow up your index finger where the large intestine meridian begins and intensify the *qi* at the webbed area of your hand between your thumb and index finger. This acupressure point is called large intestine 4 and is a key point on this meridian. Build the energy here and feel it detoxifying your body and improving the function of your large intestine. Then let the white light travel along your forearm and over to your shoulder and neck to its finishing point near the outer part of your nose. Take another deep breath through your nose and allow air to fill your lower abdomen and so stimulate your intestines. Slowly release the air ensuring that any stale residues are properly expelled. Feeling more relaxed and refreshed, with your breathing becoming deeper and steadier with every inhalation, allow the white light to flow down to your large intestine. Intensify the light and feel it cleansing your body of all the mental and physical toxins stored in your colon. Allow these to be dissolved by the white light and imagine that this then flows down your legs and out through your toes where it is transmuted by the Earth. Give thanks for this. See your body bathed in the white light. Feel peace and at one with yourself and the world.

If you wish to sleep now, stay in this deeply relaxed state of being and know that you will wake in the morning feeling refreshed and rejuvenated. If however, you want to wake, then in your own time, sense your energy becoming stronger and begin to move your fingers and toes. Take a deep breath in and feel new life and energy enter your body. Open your eyes and stretch your body out feeling yourself rejuvenated and regenerated.

# your body's own waste disposal system

## what your large intestine does for you

Bowel disorders are very prevalent today with the majority of us suffering to some degree. We should all pay more attention to the function and health of our large intestine. As with any key organ, recognizing the warning signs of imbalance and understanding their significance is crucial in preventing serious illness. Keep in mind that our waste disposal system is in truth an excellent reflection of our overall physical and emotional health. Listen to your body if you are sluggish in that department – it is essential to keep everything moving. You may find that prunes work for you, but is your body giving you a physical sign to 'let go' of old emotions attachments that are no longer needed?

### TRADITIONAL WESTERN UNDERSTANDING

Its prime function is to eliminate the by-products of digestion (the faeces) and to absorb water through the walls of the colon, so helping to conserve body fluids. The first half of this tube absorbs water from waste products, the second half acts as a storage depot for the faeces before they are expelled by the anus.

The residues of digested food empty from the small intestine into the colon in a liquid form. Peristalsis (muscular wave-like contractions of the intestine) squeezes moisture from the waste at regular intervals. This is reabsorbed back into the body and the faeces move along the length of the colon, helped by these contractions. The indigestible waste material is now relatively compact and is stored until it is time to be expelled via the anus.

The large intestine is divided into three sections: the ascending colon, transverse colon and descending colon. The ascending colon extends up the right side of the abdomen to a point near the liver (known as the hepatic flexure). From here it travels across the body (thus being termed the transverse colon) to a point on the left-hand side near the spleen (the splenic flexure). Then, like the descending colon, it travels down the left-hand side of the body, turns towards the centre of the body, leads to the rectum and finally the anus. If you ever massage your colon, always follow this natural (clockwise) direction – otherwise you will be pushing the contents the wrong way!

The appendix is another part of the colon, considered to have no real significance today by the medical profession. However, the appendix has been recognized in the East for thousands of years as playing a vital role in our immune system. This is because the appendix secretes a fluid containing anti-bacterial, antifungal and antiviral substances; this fluid also helps to lubricate the waste material, thus reducing the chance of it stagnating in the colon.

The ileocaecal valve is located at the beginning of the ascending colon and separates the small and large intestines. This can often go into spasm as a consequence of consuming certain foods that can irritate the colon such as bran. There is a correctional technique in Applied Kinesiology which is clearly outlined in the excellent book *Energy Medicine* by Donna Eden.

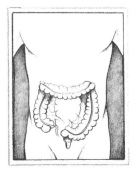

The large intestine or colon is a muscular tube about 1.5 m long. It is located in the lower abdominal region and is the last section of the digestive tract.

## TRADITIONAL CHINESE INTERPRETATION

| | |
|---|---|
| Element: | Metal |
| Partner organ: | Lungs |
| Climate: | Dryness |
| Season: | Autumn |
| Colour: | White |
| Time of day: | 5–7 a.m. |
| Body tissue: | Skin |
| Voice sound: | Weeping |
| Sense organ: | Nose |
| Reflector: | Body Hair |
| Taste: | Spicy |
| Emotion: | Grief |

## SYMPTOMS OF IMBALANCE

### Physical Symptoms

Constipation, diarrhoea • Flatulence (especially smelly wind) • Strong odours from faeces • Lower abdominal pain • Swollen colon, loss of abdominal tone •

your body's own waste disposal system

Body and foot odour • Bad breath •
Appendicitis • Diverticulitis • Haemorrhoids •
Poor memory • Skin problems: dull, dry,
flaky skin, spots etc

The large intestine continually takes in food and 'transports, transforms and eliminates'. It has a direct impact on and complementary relationship with its partner organ, the lungs, because if there is excess *qi* in the large intestine this travels upwards to the lungs.

When the colon is out of balance, the whole body is affected. Toxic wastes build up and can eventually filter back into the system. Toxins stored in the body will make the skin more coarse and your body more likely to experience aches and pains. Symptoms such as constipation, diarrhoea, flatulence and lower abdominal pain are obvious signs to watch out for. Also, abdominal distension, bad breath, haemorrhoids and poor memory can indicate a sluggish colon. There is also a close relationship between body odour and toxins in the colon. If someone, no matter how frequently they wash, cannot control their body odour and the smell of their feet, this can illustrate that the colon is not in good shape. It is not a good idea to use anti-perspirant containing aluminium as this further suppresses your body's attempt to eliminate toxins. Use natural alternatives such as deokrystal by Green People or No Offense™ by Origins. Flatulence arises when one or more of the digestive organs such as the stomach, liver, gall bladder, small intestine or pancreas is not secreting sufficient digestive juices, and can disappear when a proper diet is followed and intestinal function is restored.

## Emotional Symptoms

Inability to let go of past hurt • Melancholy • Pessimism
• Grief • Weakness and vulnerability • Cynical behaviour
• Narrow and constricted attitude

### Helping you understand more about the Mind–Body Link

The phrase 'to have the guts' to do something reflects the age-old belief that the large intestine holds sway over our courage and fortitude. When the large intestine is weak, we may not be able to fight the difficulties that face us and may lack determination, which can lead to disappointment, despair and bitterness. Just as the large intestine is continually working on waste in the body and chewing things over, the mind does the same thing psychologically. Petty behaviour, hanging on to negativity and continual dissatisfaction are some of the behaviour patterns to expect. We may become unable to appreciate anything or anyone, so can lose our family and friends and become isolated and lonely.

Grief is the emotion connected to the Metal Element; it is well known that intense grief can have a profound impact on our health and wellbeing. If we have lost someone it is perfectly natural to grieve, but there does come a time when it is essential to 'let go'. Counselling and affirmations (*see page 250*) can greatly assist in this process. Do not forget deep breathing exercises, as these will not only remove stagnant carbon dioxide but will also move blood and oxygen into the lungs – the partner of the large intestine – to release congestion. While doing deep breathing exercises, be willing to repeat affirmations about letting go of the past, and visualize any grief and pain being 'let go' by your body.

People who cannot 'let go' retain all types of unnecessary garbage as problems are kept inside – as with constipation the body holds on to old rubbish that is no longer needed. Events that have happened in our past affect our behaviour and happiness in the present. Some people like to hang on to the past and blame others for their present unhappiness, instead of taking positive, decisive action to improve matters by learning to forgive. It is the ability to forgive that is important. If we cannot forgive ourselves, this can lead to self-destructive behaviour. All we can do is learn from our experiences – to become better, kinder and more positive human beings. We need to focus on positive, uplifting, nurturing thoughts and feelings and give less power to those negative, destructive thought patterns that only serve to reduce our energy levels and destroy joy and peace of mind. Try using the 'Law of Substitution': whenever a negative message begins to play in your head, stop it in its tracks and replace it with a positive affirmation. If you are too upset and cannot even focus on an affirmation, quietly say a simple word such as 'peace' and feel calmness filling your body and soul.

# the 9 ways to health

## way 1: chinese and natural nutrition

### FOODS FOR THE METAL ELEMENT

Grain: rice
Fruit: chestnut
Meat: horse[1]
Vegetable: onions

[1]    While horse meat is recommended for this element, I do not condone its consumption.

## DIETARY TIPS

1 The most important foods for colon maintenance and cleansing are vegetables and fibre. Cellulose, the structural material of vegetables and fruit, is a very dense form of carbohydrate which has the ability to stimulate and enhance the function of the intestine. With all the curves and bends in the intestine, wastes can become lodged, creating pockets in the bowels (known as diverticulitis) where bacteria can flourish. We have forgotten how to feed our colons, they have been made redundant with all the fast and refined foods that are part of the nineties diet. Many medical researchers believe that cancer and other diseases of the colon can be prevented with a diet containing large amounts of vegetable fibre. Fibre is needed to speed the expulsion process in the colon; if absent from the diet, colon contents stagnate and the disease process can begin.

2 Foods that contain a high proportion of water are also important, as are those with either a neutral pH or an alkaline pH. This is because our body's acid-alkaline balance is often 80 per cent acid/20 per cent alkaline when it should ideally be 80 per cent alkaline/20 per cent acid! Vegetables are wonderfully alkaline foods, so include them in abundance in your diet, and especially if you suffer from problems with the large intestine. The exceptions are members of the nightshade family of vegetables – potatoes, tomatoes, aubergines, peppers, as well as tobacco – which contain a toxin called solanine to which individuals suffering from body pain and arthritis are very sensitive. Citrus fruits are also best avoided by those sensitive individuals whose digestive system cannot tolerate anything too acidic.

3 In Chinese Medicine, raw food is seen to weaken the spleen. This can make the body more prone to being 'cold and damp' with symptoms such as water retention, slightly sticky hands, abdominal distension and loose stools. If you are really hooked on raw food, then at least create some balance by warming your body up with

herbs such as ginger and cinnamon. See the chapter on the spleen (*page 68*) for other food recommendations. Unless you already consume large amounts of raw foods, start slowly and gently with any cleansing programme. Raw fruit and honey are especially 'aggressive' cleansers. Some vegetables also have a strong cleansing action, so these too are best eaten in moderation in the early stages – onions, leeks, chives, fenugreek and turnips.

4  For the average person, this is not always the best way to start a cleansing programme as it can swing the body into 'shock cleansing'. This is because toxins are stored in the body in the deep organs such as the liver and kidneys. When you go on to a raw cleansing diet, the toxins are brought up from these organs to the superficial systems of elimination, where the bowel, skin and lymphatic system all play crucial roles. However, if these systems have not been prepared in advance for such a cleansing, it can put considerable strain on the organs in the body and trigger a 'healing crisis'. A cleansing reaction or healing crisis occurs when toxic substances are expelled from the body tissues faster than the organs of elimination can remove them, leading to toxicity in the blood and lymph.

5  The Chinese believe that eating more refined foods and fewer fibre and vegetables causes us to have less *qi*. Toxins build up inside the body and begin to poison our system by a process known as 'auto-intoxication' where the body reabsorbs toxins from the waste lying in the colon. This affects the liver and symptoms can include anything from mood changes and irritability to more chronic conditions. The blood is also affected, as the liver's filtering job is impaired, which can have a negative effect on the whole body.

6  Air pollution, smoking and central heating and travelling also contribute to dehydration and thus constipation. It is essential, therefore, to drink plenty of water. Remember, in the colder months, to drink warm water and avoid ice water if possible.

**Foods that strengthen the Colon and Metal Element**

*(also see Recipes, page 289)*:

❋ Aduki beans, aubergines, bean curd, cauliflower, celery, Chinese cabbage, corn, cucumber, figs, honey, lettuce, onions and yellow soya beans are some of the foods recommended by traditional Chinese medicine to support the colon.

❋ Increase consumption of grains such as rice and millet. Millet is a gluten-free, alkaline grain which does not create mucus in the body. However, it can be very stodgy if not prepared correctly. Soak it overnight and rinse well, then simmer for 10 minutes, watching carefully that it doesn't get too thick. It does have a rather bland taste (that's putting it politely!) and is best added to flavoursome soups or tossed into a stir-fry with plenty of garden herbs.

❋ Increase your vegetable intake: steam or stir-fry them with seaweed and spices such as ginger and garlic. Try vegetable soups. You can stir-fry without oil – sweat an onion in a small amount of water. Once the onion has released its juices, add spices and herbs, followed by the vegetables.

❋ Avocado, sprouting seeds and pulses make excellent and highly nutritious ingredients in any meal.

❋ Eat only moderate amounts of animal protein (meat and poultry) if you are very constipated, as it can slow down the process of peristalsis in the intestine. Make vegetables and rice the main part of your meals, with meat as a 'side dish'.

❋ Flax seed or linseed is also excellent as it not only delivers essential fatty acids but is a superb lubricant which can help to heal and repair inflamed tubes. You can buy raw linseeds (dark brown in colour) or a product called Linseed Gold, which is grown organically. You must chew these very well or soak overnight or you can buy flax oil, Udo's Choice being an excellent organic product rich in omega 3 and 6 essential fatty acids. Ensure that these products are kept in a fridge or freezer to keep them from going rancid.

**Foods that weaken the Colon and Metal Element:**

※ Avoid wheat bran, as it can scratch the lining of the large intestine. Whole grain oats are a better source of fibre and are kinder on the colon. Wheat bran is also high in a substance known as phytate or phytic acid, which has the capacity to bind to minerals such as calcium and magnesium, thus preventing the body from absorbing them. The absorption of zinc and iron may also be impaired in this way.

※ Milk and dairy products are not viewed as particularly beneficial to the colon as they can bring on diarrhoea and vomiting in susceptible individuals and contribute towards congestion. If you are not sensitive to dairy products, the addition of live natural yoghurt (made from either cow's, goat's or sheep's milk) can replenish the amount of the valuable lactobacillus acido philus bacteria in the colon, so helping to keep levels of putrefactive bacteria down.

※ Pomegranates can be very irritating to the colon and should be avoided. Nuts should not be eaten if you suffer from diverticulitis.

※ Cocoa, tea and coffee contain caffeine which can contribute to gastric troubles, ulcers and indigestion. The aromatic oils in coffee can cause diarrhoea; the tannin in tea induces constipation. Tea, coffee, chocolate, soft drinks and alcohol are diuretics, removing fluids and minerals from the body and causing dehydration.

※ Soya beans are mucus-forming and intake should be limited. However, if the beans are sprouted for six days they lose their mucus properties.


## way 2: herbs and spices

※ The Ayurvedic formula Triphala can be taken at night as it stimulates 'peristalsis' – wave-like contractions of the colon that encourage your body to properly rid itself of the contents. An organic version is available from Healing Herb Supplies (UK).

※ Basil is helpful for constipation.

❋ Ginger root, black pepper, nutmeg, garlic, mustard greens and daikon radish are medicinal herbs for the Metal Element.

❋ Psyllium husks are classically used in bowel formulae as they swell with water, forming a wallpaper-like solution, and are unsurpassed at loosening old matter and increasing the size of the bulky mass travelling though the intestine. However, it is of a 'cool' nature according to food energetics; some vitamin companies such as Biocare UK have now started to add herbs such as ginger to 'warm up' these formulae.

❋ Aloe vera juice cleanses, heals and soothes the bowel and is excellent for inflammatory bowel disorders. However, it is of a 'cool' nature, so cold individuals must ensure that their diet includes 'warming' foods to compensate.

❋ Slippery elm too has excellent healing properties as it coats the inner membranes of the digestive tract, thus allowing healing of the underlying tissues to take place.

❋ Herbal Elixir by Green People is a synergistic combination of 16 organically grown, cold-pressed herbs including nettles, ginger and dandelion and is designed to eliminate toxins and help flush your colon.

## way 3: exercise

Too much lying down can damage the lung and large intestine meridians, affecting both elimination and respiration. To remedy this, work on acu-pressure point Large Intestine 4, located in the muscle between the thumb and first finger, and on Large Intestine 11, found at the elbow crease on the outer part of the arm (*see diagram, page 247*). While these points are being stimulated, make the lung sound 'SSSSS' and visualize the colour white healing and decongesting your large intestine.

An exercise to stretch the large intestine and lung meridians is described on *page 221*.

Deep breathing and relaxation exercises are very important to help re-educate the bowel. Remember that the lungs are the partner organ to the large intestine, so deep breathing will always have a positive impact on the bowels. See the exercises recommended on *page 222*.

## way 4: massage and reflex points

Massaging the large intestine can be very therapeutic and helps to clear away some of the deposits that have built up over the years. Use an olive oil cream, or olive oil from the kitchen, to which a few drops of the essential oils recommended (*page 248*) have been added.

When undertaking any colon massage, it is important to drain the descending colon first, which is on the left-hand side.

❋ Start by placing your hand just beneath your spleen on the left-hand side of your body. Using the heel of your hand, gently glide over the colon, feeling for any lumps and bumps. Passing the inside of the left hip bone, gently draw your hand towards your pubic bone. Repeat three times.

❋ Move your hand to the liver region on the right-hand side, just beneath your ribs. Again, using the heel of your hand, gently glide it across to the left-hand side, noting any bumpy patches, and down the descending colon as described in Step 1. Repeat three times.

❋ Now move to the lowest point of the ascending colon, on the inside right hip. Glide the heel of your hand up towards the liver, three times.

❋ Going back to the lowest point of the ascending colon, slide your hand up towards the liver area, across to the spleen, down the left hip and gently across to the pubic bone. Repeat three times.

❋ Use your fingers to massage the whole colon area in a circular motion, following the (clockwise) direction of the colon, for a further two times. At this stage you can pay a little more attention to the knotted areas of the colon by massaging in small circles directly over them, moving on when they feel a little looser. This will begin to move the energy in the intestine and help relieve constipation.

Remember that your colon may have taken many years to get into its current state, so don't expect it to be clear after just a few sessions! You may notice that your bowel motions appear darker than usual. This just means that the old wastes that have built up and stuck to the walls of your intestine have been loosened and released. (However, if you see blood in your stool, consult your GP.)

There is also an extra area that is excellent to massage, if somewhat painful! The *fascia lata* muscle is located on the outside of the thigh from the knee to the top of the thigh, where the side seam of trousers would run. This is the neuro-lymphatic point for the large intestine according to Applied Kinesiology. It will probably feel both tender and lumpy to the touch, but gently massaging this area with oil, or even just rubbing it through your trousers when you have a spare moment, will help to support the function of the large intestine. Skin brushing is an excellent way to help detoxify your body. For techniques and information, refer to page 77.

The colon is one of the more complicated reflexology zones to massage as you must start on the left foot and work on the ileo-caecal valve and ascending colon, across half of the transverse colon, and continue on to the right foot, still following the transverse colon until you move on to the descending colon and rectum. One easy-to-follow method is to massage this reflex in tiny circular movements (noting particularly 'gritty' areas), gradually working along the length of the colon. When you have completed this, you can return to the trouble spots and gently massage these again. (*See page 23 for massage techniques.*)

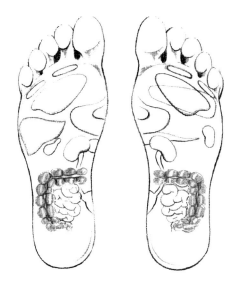

*Reflexology Points for the Large Intestine (shaded)*

## way 5: acupressure

The large intestine meridian begins at the outside tip of the index finger and travels to Large Intestine 4, a major point located in the webbing between the thumb and the index finger. It runs along the forearm and up to the shoulder and, after dividing into two channels, finishes at the nose. To trace the meridian, start at the outside tip of your index finger and run your palm along your forearm to the shoulder. Run towards your neck, up to your nose and finish on the outside at the flair of your nose.

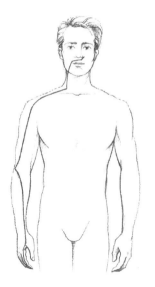

*The Large Intestine Meridian*

### Large Intestine 4

This is a key point on the large intestine meridian, but should **not** be used on pregnant women. It is a valuable point that can help to detoxify the body by relieving constipation and improving the function of the large intestine. It is a good point to help improve the complexion. It can also relieve frontal headaches, shoulder pain and toothache. Good to massage when you are watching television!

### Large Intestine 11

To find this point, bend your elbow and take your thumb along the crease until you feel a slight depression before the bone. It will probably be tender! This is an effective point to massage to relieve constipation and stimulate a sluggish bowel. It is also a good point to foster a blooming complexion, especially if used in conjunction with LI 4.

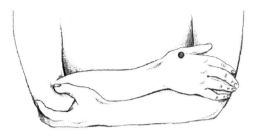

*Large Intestine 4 and 11 Acupressure Points*

## way 6: essential oils

**Fennel:** rebalances the digestive system and stimulates the flow of energy in the large intestine, so helping with bloating and flatulence. Its antispasmodic properties can release tension held in the intestines. Encourages us to communicate and show our feelings rather than allowing them to fester. *Strength factor: Strong*

**German chamomile:** heals inflammation in the bowel, making it useful for diarrhoea and general bowel symptoms such as irritable bowel disease. If the cause of diarrhoea is an allergy to a certain food, this oil would be a good choice due to its calming, soothing and antispasmodic properties. *Strength factor: Strong*

**Thyme:** primarily known for its action on the lungs, but it also has an antiseptic and anti-fungal effect on the large intestine so can be useful in the treatment of candidiasis and intestinal worms. Helps to ease complaints such as sluggish digestion, abdominal distension and flatulence.

**Tea tree:** a powerful disinfectant oil with anti-fungal, anti-biotic and anti-viral properties which is often selected as an oil of choice for problems such as candidiasis, intestinal parasites or skin infections. It is also thought to calm inflammation of the intestines. *Strength factor: Strong*

If you have dry skin or eczema ensure that you take essential fatty acids (*page 16*) and regularly apply an oil blend to your skin that is nourishing and contains no irritants. Good products include Calming Composition™ by Aveda which contains many soothing flower and plant essences including rose and Body Wisdom Organics Metal Element Elixir. Origins do a spray to put on damp skin called Birthday Suit™ which is ideal for sensitive skin and a warming one which includes ginger called Ginger Gloss™. Bathing in Dead Sea Salts (*see page 148 in Kidney chapter or Water Element section*) is also highly beneficial.

If your stools are loose and you frequently suffer from diarrhoea, it is important to consider the possible causes. It could be too much cold food, nerves, allergies or parasites. If it has been triggered by a virus or bacterial infection, then **Eucalyptus** and **Tea Tree** oils would be most helpful. However, for stress-induced bowel problems brought on by excessive workloads, exams or an interview, for example, anti-spasmodic oils such as **Lavender** and **Neroli** can be used. The latter is especially good as a pre-ventative to help alleviate stress and anxiety before they lead to diarrhoea. If there is much pain and cramp due to spasm of the intestinal muscles, try oil of **Ginger** combined with **Fennel**, as both are warming and carmi-native oils. Oil of **Rosemary** is an excellent bowel stimulant.

## way 7: flower remedies

**Crab Apple:** known as the cleansing remedy. For those wishing to purify the body. Indicated when there are feelings of being 'unclean': Dr Bach described it as 'the remedy which helps us to get rid of anything we do not like either in our minds or bodies'. Helps us to process negativity, impurities and unresolved issues.

**Honeysuckle:** for when your life has got 'stuck in the past'. For those who romanticize over past times and are nostalgic, often missing the present times as they are so preoccupied with dwelling on the past. Focuses the mind on the here and now so we can learn to put the past into its proper perspective.

**Pine:** for those who carry feelings of guilt, often when the wrongdoing is not of their own making. Initiates the process of forgiveness and invokes feelings of genuine regret rather than guilt.

**Walnut:** known as the 'link breaker', helping to break negative thought patterns and encouraging us to let go, move on and cultivate more positive and nourishing thoughts. Dr Bach called it 'the remedy for those who have decided to take a great step forward in life, to break old conventions, to leave old limits and restrictions and start on a new way'.

**Red Chrysanthemum:** FF19 is the bowel formula that is used for constipation, stagnation of the colon, Irritable Bowel Syndrome and diarrhoea. Emotionally, it is for those who cannot let go and who cling to the past and situations that really need to be released.

Alternatively, try the Phytobiophysics Large Intestine Meridian Formula or the Metal Element Flower Formula by Body Wisdom Organics.

You may also find some appropriate flower remedies for supporting the Metal Element in the chapter on the lungs (*page 228*).

## way 8: affirmations

- ❋ I trust my large intestine to eliminate all waste products from my body easily.
- ❋ I now forgive myself and others, so enabling me to move forward in life.
- ❋ My skin covers and protects my whole body and is healthy, clear and glowing.

✳ It is safe for me to process and release anything that is no longer needed by my mind, body and spirit.

*See also the Lungs chapter, page 230, for affirmations that may be used in conjunction with these.*

## way 9: meditation for soul nourishment

*See Lungs chapter, page 230.*

# taking a deeper look
# at chinese medicine

Traditional Chinese Medicine (TCM) is a system of diagnosis and healthcare which has evolved over the last 4,000 years and is a unique approach to understanding the human body. In Chinese medicine, health is viewed as a totally complete state of wellbeing, which is a different approach to Western medicine, which defines health as merely the 'absence of disease'.

The *Huang Ti Nei Jing*, or *Yellow Emperor's Classic of Internal Medicine*, is a corpus of writings on Chinese Medicine. There are several versions, some of which no longer exist. The most commonly known was compiled by Wang Ping during the Tang dynasty. It was an intellectual tradition which started in the 2nd–3rd centuries BC. It was considered then, as it is today, to be an indispensable treatise on acupuncture, and an important reference material for the study and practice of Traditional Chinese Medicine (TCM). While back in the 2nd century BC it reflected current beliefs and practices, it also claimed to draw on ancient sources dating back a further 3,000 years when people were said to have experienced high levels of health and greater longevity.

TCM is based on the belief that all humanity is part of the natural environment and that health or balance can only be achieved when one follows the natural law, adapting to the changes of the seasons and the surrounding environment. This is the philosophy of the *dao*, and the Chinese believed (and still do today) that the more we stray from living in harmony with the *dao*, the more certain it is that no form of external medicine or treatment could ever compensate for the stresses that will affect the mind, body and spirit. The theories of *yin* and *yang*, together with the notion of the five elements, were developed through ancient Chinese rituals of observing nature's ever changing cycles. These theories are fundamental to Chinese Medicine.

## the five elements

The five elements are Wood, Fire, Earth, Metal and Water. These are related to the different seasons of the year and to organs in the human body. By knowing and understanding these elements, we can discover how to balance the extremes of each season and comprehend what unique opportunities for growth arise with each. The organs are interlinked with the seasons, temperatures, colours and tastes, to name but a few associations, all of which have some relevance to our health and wellbeing. The five element theory shows the interrelationship of the organs in a very general way. However, it is essential to understand that the relationships between the different organs can be very complex. Sometimes it may be that one element is out of balance, but when disease is chronic it is very likely that all of the key organs could be affected to a greater or lesser degree.

The Wood phase occurs in Spring, which is a time in nature of activity and new beginnings. This is followed by the Fire Element in Summer, which is the season of abundance where the ideas that were put into action in the Spring have blossomed and flowered. The Earth phase arrives in late Summer and is the harvest season, a time when we can reap the benefits of the seeds planted in the early Spring. Metal is connected with Autumn, the time of decline when nature slowly begins to withdraw in preparation for the Winter. The life force in nature lies dormant during the Winter months of the Water Element, like the latent seed that is lying still and waiting to burst open in the Spring to begin the cycle once again. (See table on *page 273*.)

## sheng and ko cycles

The five elements are often depicted as illustrated in the diagram below, which shows how the organs are all interrelated and can demonstrate how an imbalance in one element will have a corresponding effect on the other elements within the cycle. There are two important cycles in the five element theory: the *Sheng*, or generation cycle, and the *Ko*, or controlling cycle.

### GENERATION, OR SHENG CYCLE

*Qi* (or life-force) travels round from element to element:

- ☀ **Water** nourishes the plants and trees, generating **Wood**.
- ☀ **Wood** can be burned to generate **Fire**.
- ☀ **Fire** leaves behind ashes that are absorbed into the **Earth**.
- ☀ **Earth** contains the ores that form **Metal**.
- ☀ **Metal** (mineral ores) enrich the **Water**.

There is another way of interpreting this cycle, which is to substitute the elements for the key organs (these are known in Chinese medicine as the *yin* organs). So, when Water nourishes Wood, the kidney, which is the *yin* organ of the Water Element, helps to feed the liver and strengthen its energy. By strengthening the liver (Wood), blood is generated which is stored in this organ. Blood is needed by the *yin* organ of the Fire Element,

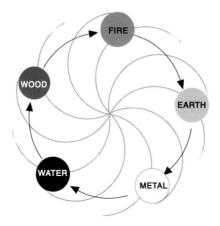

*The Sheng Cycle*

the heart, so the liver plays a supporting role to the heart. The fiery energy of the heart supports the spleen, the *yin* organ of the Earth Element, by supplying the necessary heat and energy to assist the spleen in its function of processing food. The spleen then nurtures Metal by taking the resultant food essence upwards and combining this with the air from the lungs to form pure *qi*. The lungs, the *yin* organ of the Metal Element, then play a supporting role to the kidneys by sending moist *qi* or energy to be stored in the kidneys. Diseases where there is weakness or 'deficiency' (as it is known in TCM) tend to follow the path of the *Sheng* cycle, where the weak 'child' draws heavily on its 'mother' for support, so draining her reserves.

## MOTHER AND CHILD RELATIONSHIP

This is sometimes expressed as the law of the Mother and Child. One way to interpret this is to imagine a simple family scenario. When a mother has a baby and breastfeeds her, if there are any illnesses with the mother, it affects the quality of her milk. This then will have a corresponding effect on the child, who will become sick as she is not receiving adequate nutrition. The other possibility with this law is that the child could be particularly hungry and so deplete the mother by drawing too heavily on her supplies, leading to the mother becoming ill. The mother's role is to ensure that the child's and her own vital needs are met.

Building the organs into the picture, a good example to use is the liver as the mother and the heart as the child. When the 'mother' (the liver) is sick, it will affect the flow of *qi* to the 'child' (the heart). This means that the 'child' could start to produce symptoms such as palpitations, anxiety and chest pains.

Frequently in Western medicine, the first reaction is to treat the immediate obvious symptoms of disease. However, if we could only look a little further and find out *why* the body has produced symptoms, then perhaps we could learn to treat the cause of the problem instead of merely its symptoms. This is the importance of understanding where the 'mother' of a disease lies. In the example given above, treating the heart alone would not be the most suitable route to take, as the original cause in this instance stems from the liver. By treating the true cause of the imbalance, you will re-establish harmony in all the related organs.

## CHART OF MOTHER AND CHILD RELATIONSHIPS

| Mother | Child |
|---|---|
| Wood (liver) | Fire (heart) |
| Fire (heart) | Earth (spleen) |
| Earth (spleen) | Metal (lungs) |
| Metal (lungs) | Water (kidneys) |
| Water (kidneys) | Wood (liver) |

## CONTROLLING, OR KO CYCLE

The controlling or *Ko* cycle applies constraints to the relationships between various elements:

taking a deeper look at chinese medicine

- ❋ **Wood** can deplete the **Earth** of its nutrients.
- ❋ **Earth** absorbs **Water**, channelling and containing it.
- ❋ **Water** can overcome **Fire**.
- ❋ **Fire** can melt **Metal**.
- ❋ **Metal** controls **Wood** (as metal tools can cut through trees).

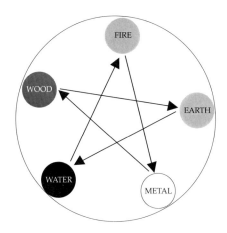

*The Ko Cycle*

In organ terms, we may see a disease beginning, for example, in the Wood Element (the liver). If the problem goes undetected, it will affect the spleen and digestion (Earth), which then go on to imbalance the kidney (Water). The next element in the *Ko* cycle is Fire, so we see the disharmony going on to affect the heart and then the lung (Metal). It is interesting to note the correlation of the heart and kidneys when the *Ko* cycle follows a destructive path: this is confirmed in Western medicine when excessive fluid retention weakens the heart and diuretics are prescribed.

# emotions

Today, Western medicine is at long last beginning to validate the healing power not only of the body, but of the mind. Exciting research has transformed our concept of the mind and it is now thought that the mind has a presence throughout the entire body. This is because the cells which carry emotions in the brain have recently been discovered to exist in our immune system. The Chinese have understood for thousands of years that our thoughts and emotions have a great impact on the state of our health and that emotional distress compromises the health of the body.

There are five emotions, which are connected to the five elements and to the major *yin* organs (the liver, heart, spleen, lungs and kidneys). Anger relates to the liver, joy to the heart, pensiveness to the spleen, grief to the lungs and fear to the kidneys. Extremes of emotions can have a negative impact on the organs, especially when they are intense or have been suppressed for some time, just as an imbalanced organ can have a profound effect on the state of our emotions.

## EARTH

Worry or sympathy are the emotions connected to the Earth Element. Sympathy can display itself at times when we are over-sympathetic to circumstances or, alternatively, cannot bear people fussing over us. Someone who continually seeks as much sympathy as possible, the individual who happily tells you all about their health problems and woes, or who is constantly worrying, has an imbalance in the spleen or stomach.

## WOOD

Excessive amounts of anger or feelings of frustration, irritation or suppressed rage point to the Wood Element and show us that it is not functioning harmoniously. The Chinese, however, readily admit there are appropriate times for expressing anger and it is better to vent our feelings rather than to seethe and suppress this powerful emotion.

## FIRE

Laughter and joy are valuable emotions and today there is sadly not enough of these wonderful emotions on display. Someone who can't laugh or show love and affection, or who demonstrates excess amounts, reveals a Fire imbalance.

## WATER

Fear is a very real emotion and without it we might not realize when we are in dangerous situations. It can, however, consume us and this is when it is damaging to the Water Element.

## METAL

Finally, grief too is an important emotion that we experience when we go through the loss of something special. If there is an imbalance in the Metal Element, the grieving process can be prolonged beyond its natural term.

## yin and yang

Traditional Chinese medicine holds that the material world is in a constant state of flux due to the movement of *yin* and *yang*, two opposing elements which are mutually dependent (that is, they cannot exist without one another). The theory of *yin* and *yang* is used to help explain the physiological imbalances and any pathological changes in the human body. The resulting information is then used for diagnostic purposes. All the major organs in the body are paired according to the principles of *yin* and *yang* and with one of the five elements.

*Yin*, translated literally, means the 'dark side of the mountain' and represents qualities such as darkness, coldness, stillness, etc. *Yang* is translated as the 'bright side of the mountain', representing light, warmth and activity. In the chart below, *yin* and *yang* are broken down into four categories which can help to clarify and illustrate some of the roles these two opposites play in life.

| Yang | Yin |
|---|---|
| **In nature** | |
| Spring/Summer | Autumn/Winter |
| East/South | West/North |
| Day | Night |
| Hot | Cold |
| Fire | Water |
| Light | Dark |
| Sun | Moon |
| | |
| **In our bodies** | |
| Male | Female |
| Energy | Blood |
| Surfaces of the body | Internal parts of the body |
| Back of the body | Front of the body |
| Upper body | Lower body |
| Right side of the body | Left side of the body |
| | |
| **In ill-health** | |
| Acute symptoms | Chronic disease |
| Heat and high temperature | Cold and low temperature |
| Dryness | Moistness |

**Organs/meridians**

| | |
|---|---|
| Gall Bladder | Liver |
| Small intestine | Heart |
| Stomach | Spleen |
| Large intestine | Lungs |
| Bladder | Kidneys |
| *triple warmer* | *pericardium* |

## the eight principles

There are four opposing diagnostic considerations in Traditional Chinese Medicine which help the practitioner to understand the true nature of a disease or imbalance:

1   Interior and exterior
2   Heat and cold
3   Excess and deficiency
4   Yin and yang

There are many combinations of these patterns, which are too complex to explain in detail in a book of this nature. However, we can look briefly at each individual pairing:

**Interior and exterior** patterns can help to explain the aetiology of an illness – in other words, where it has come from and where in the body it actually resides. Interior diseases may be of an emotional origin (that is, caused by prolonged grief, fear, anger, etc.) and tend to develop slowly. They are more chronic and long-standing than exterior illnesses. An exterior disease tends to be more of an acute nature, brought on by external causes known as the 'six pernicious influences': Heat, Summer Heat, Dryness, Wind, Cold and Damp. You will see later in this book that these influences are connected with the elements and organs. For example, too much cold can injure the kidney/Water Element, too much heat can injure the heart/Fire Element (*see table on page 273*). If the body and *qi* are strong, you are less likely to be susceptible to these external influences. However, when there is an imbalance in the body and a weakness or deficiency of *qi*, you are more likely to contract an illness.

**Heat and cold** are used primarily to describe whether the body has symptoms of either a 'cold' nature – for example, low body temperature, pale complexion, pale urine, loose stools and a desire for hot drinks and a warm environment – or a 'hot' nature – the person will very often feel hot, look red in the face, have a thirst for cold liquids, crave fresh air or cold temperatures, and have dark urine and constipation. This information will guide the practitioner towards a suitable treatment: for example, someone showing symptoms of a cold nature will be prescribed warming herbs and warming foods. Raw foods and cold liquids would not be deemed suitable for illnesses of this nature, as the stomach has to warm the cold food, using up more *qi* to digest it and ultimately weakening the individual further.

**Excess and deficiency** is an extremely important differentiation in Chinese medicine and can demonstrate the impact that an illness is having on the body. If the patient is already weak, then he or she is likely to exhibit further deficiency symptoms (such as fatigue, loss of appetite, a soft voice and lassitude). Conversely, someone showing signs of excess will display hyper- or over-activity of body functions, such as heavy breathing and a loud voice. As the latter type is ultimately stronger, he or she will have sufficient *qi* to generate a strong reaction to the pathogen and is therefore more likely to present more obvious, visible symptoms. The important point to be made here is that the 'excess' patient may show more marked signs of illness, but the 'deficient' patient may be in a more critical state, and care must be taken to ensure that he or she does not become weakened further.

*Yin* and *yang*, as discussed earlier, are fundamental to TCM. They encompass the six influences above: your practitioner when making a diagnosis will check to see what imbalances you have and whether they could be defined as interior or exterior, hot or cold, excess or deficient. This will help the practitioner to understand and determine the *yin/yang* disharmony in your body.

## essential substances

There are various substances that are considered to be essential in Chinese Medicine which help to nourish all levels of our being. I have outlined below the five fundamental substances: *Jing* (essence), *Shen* (spirit), *Xue* (blood), *Qi* (life-force) and *Jin Ye* (body fluids).

### JING

We are all born with this special prenatal essence or *Jing* which we inherit from our parents and which, in many respects, helps to define our basic constitution. Children born of healthy parents will have a strong essence or *Jing*, whereas children whose parents have a weaker constitution will often have inherited less. *Jing* is discussed in more depth in the chapter on the kidneys (*page 148*), as the kidneys store the *Jing*.

### SHEN

The *Shen* or spirit resides in the heart which, according to the principles of Chinese medicine, is often seen as the organ most connected with heaven. The concept of the *Shen* is a complex one, as there are many interpretations. It is probably best translated as 'spirit', although some authorities interpret it as the mind. More information on the *Shen* is found in the chapter on the heart (*page 89*).

## XUE

The blood (*Xue*) plays a vital role in both Western and Chinese medicine. The Chinese believe that blood travels not only in the blood vessels, but also in the meridians or energy channels of the body. It is classified as a *yin* substance.

## JIN YE

*Jin Ye* pertains to all the other body fluids and secretions – saliva, synovial fluid (lubricates the joints) and mucus. Oedema (water retention) illustrates an imbalance in body fluids.

## QI

*Qi* or *chi* (pronounced 'chee') can be translated as 'vital energy' or life-force, but even these words do not capture what *qi* really is. It has been described as the force that nourishes both the body and mind, and the free-flow of this vital energy around the body is seen as imperative to our health and wellbeing. If the *qi* becomes imbalanced, or there is a blockage (*stagnation*), there is too little (a *deficiency*) or even too much (*excess*), disease can result. The flow of this vital energy can be impeded by poor diet, lack of exercise, poor breathing and posture, scar tissue and psychological stress.

*Qi* flows through the body in pathways called *meridians*.

## the meridian system

The meridians are channels that carry the *qi* around the body. The ancient Chinese philosophy of energy is referred to as the meridian system. Diagrams dating back to 3000 BC have been discovered on walls of caves depicting the flow of energy through these meridians. This ancient system has been used for centuries to heal and treat a broad range of imbalances in the body. The meridian channels act rather like the circulatory system which ensures that the blood travels throughout your body and can be likened to an 'energy' bloodstream. Although in modern society we use more electrical technology than ever before, in the West we still remain suspicious and sceptical of the vital importance of free flowing energy through our bodies for health. Thus the importance of electrical or energetic medicine has never really been fully understood or respected. There are 12 major organ meridians and eight extra channels. Both acupuncture and acupressure work on specific points along the meridians called acupuncture points. If these are congested it can impede the energy flow, possibly resulting in pain or problems in the associated organ. Meridians are a useful means of detecting imbalances in the organs well in advance of more chronic problems developing. Working on chosen points on the meridian can help to redirect and circulate the energy to the organs that need it, thus establishing harmony in our system.

Phytobiophysics, developed by Dame Diana Mossop (*see page 6*) is a powerful new scientific philosophy designed to treat the complex health problems of modern society by utilizing the energetic properties of plants to restore the correct flow of energy through the meridian system of the human body. The fourteen Phytobiophysics Meridian Flower formulas have been compiled as a result of many years of alchemy and research into combining the different energies of plants and are designed to tune the meridians and restore optimum function. Our combined effort has produced a powerful range of potent remedies that draw on the strength of flower formulas as well as a range of flower essence blends by Body Wisdom Organics which combines specific Phytobiophysics meridian formulas to bring balance to each of the five elements. These powerful meridian flower essences are contained in an organic herbal or flower tincture to allow a resonance with the physical body and organs.

There are 12 major meridians, two of which are not covered in detail in this book are the *pericardium* and the *triple warmer/burner*. These are not linked to physical organs in a sense, but have very important roles to play in health. The *pericardium* is known as the 'heart protector' whose key function is to stop anything harmful from reaching the heart. It is thought to take the brunt of physical and emotional pressure.

The *triple warmer* regulates the temperature of the internal organs and has a connection to our thyroid gland that ensures we have a healthy metabolism. The *triple warmer* (*san jiao*) is the method by which the *Jin Ye* or body fluids move from one organ function to another. Another interpretation maintains that the *triple warmer* regulates the temperature of the internal organs, ensuring they are kept within their ideal range. It is the only channel which traverses the body in a spiral fashion, rather than a straight line.

The *triple warmer* is divided into three sections: the upper warmer, which consists of the lungs, heart and *pericardium*; the middle warmer, which consists of the digestive organs; and the lower warmer, which contains the remaining organs of elimination as well as the kidneys and liver. However, some TCM practitioners consider the liver to be in the middle warmer. The phytobiophysics formula FF9 Bluebell is designed to support the triple energiser and thyroid and the two meridians are included in the Body Wisdom Organics Fire Element Flower Formula.

There are also eight Extra Meridians that include the Conception vessel (also known as the *yin* or central meridian) and the Governing vessel (or *yang* meridian) yet only these two are considered to be major meridians as they both have specific meridian points unlike the other six Extra Meridians. The Phytobiophysics formula FF1 activates the pineal master controller and supports the Governor vessel and FF2 is the formula for the Conception vessel.

## the organs

The *yin* organs are also called the 'zang' organs; they are solid organs involved primarily with collecting and storing, whereas the *yang* or 'fu' organs are hollow, more involved in transforming and transporting. When disharmony affecting the organs is brought back into balance as much as possible, diseases of the mind and body subside.

## tongue and pulse diagnosis

These two diagnostic techniques play a fundamental role in Traditional Chinese Medicine. It is not appropriate to describe either method in depth here, as they have to be carried out by a trained practitioner. Suffice to say that pulse diagnosis bears no resemblance to the physical examination of the pulse carried out in Western medicine; the latter is primarily concerned with the speed of the pulse. TCM focuses on the quality of the pulse in six different positions, three positions on each wrist at a superficial or deep level. Acupuncturists also can detect imbalances from a medial position. The *yin* organs are felt at a deep level and the *yang* organs at a superficial level. On the left wrist you find the heart, liver and kidney at the deep level and their *yang* counterpart organs, small intestine, gall bladder and bladder, at the superficial level. The right pulses denote the lung, spleen and *pericardium yin* organs and superficial positions reflect the large intestine, stomach and *triple warmer*.

In tongue diagnosis, a practitioner assesses the condition of the tongue, observing in particular the colour, texture (wet, dry, shiny, sticky, etc.), shape and any coating on the body of the tongue. These characteristics may vary in different sections of the tongue, which correspond to the organs of the body.

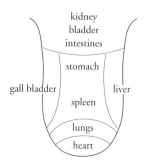

*Tongue Diagnosis*

## moxibustion

Moxibustion is the process of burning the herb Mugwort (Moxa) over certain areas of the body (including acupressure points) to increase internal warmth and energy both in the meridians and throughout the body. Mugwort (*Artemisia vulgaris latiflora*) has the ability to transfer heat generated by burning a moxa stick approximately 2.5 cm away from the desired location on the body. It is an excellent preventative as well as a tonic, as it regulates, nourishes and moves the *qi* and can also warm it if we are cold. Burning Moxa over acupressure point Stomach 36 is an excellent way of increasing energy – the Chinese recommend that everyone over 30 does this (*see page 57*). Burning it over Bladder 23 also increases energy and supports the kidneys (*see page 140*). If there is no movement or warmth in the lower burner, it is good to burn moxa over points CV 4 and 6 (*see diagram overleaf*).

At the *very* first signs of a cold or flu, moxa LI 4 (*see page 248*) for five minutes, on each hand – this will help stop the cold or flu from developing, but only if done immediately you feel the symptoms coming on.
**WARNING:** Never use moxibustion on an area where there is a lot of heat or congestion. Other contraindications include fever, high blood pressure, diabetes or sensitive skin.

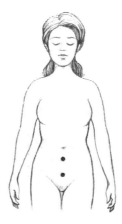

*CV 4 (below) and 6 (above)*

## TECHNIQUE

Moxa is best applied by using a moxa stick, which looks rather like a large cigar (can be purchased from a Chinese pharmacy). Peel the top coloured wrapper and light the stick, allowing it to burn until it produces some smoke. Holding the stick like a pencil with your hand halfway up its length, place the burning tip approximately 2.5 cm above the chosen acupressure point or area. Feel the warmth increasing – when it becomes too hot, withdraw the stick for a few moments. Briefly touch the point with your hand to cool the skin, then reapply the heat using a 'pecking' technique: hold the tip close until you cannot tolerate any more heat, then pull it away. Alternatively, you can move the stick slowly in a clockwise direction over the affected area. Continue for several minutes until you feel that the heat has truly penetrated the area and warmed it up. To extinguish, cut off the oxygen to the stick by stubbing it out in a jar of salt or sand, or wrap it in foil, or place it upside down into a long metal candlestick holder (never hold it under water).

## lifestyle

Our lifestyle and its effects on our health are very important factors in Chinese medicine, especially in the areas of diet, exercise and sexual activity. Diet is an important factor in most cultures and the Chinese are no different; Chinese diets are, in a sense, more holistic and primarily designed to heal many common ailments, from constipation and diarrhoea to colds or skin disorders. The Chinese approach is far more complete than the Western one, as it dates back to the time before foods were classified according to their protein, fat, carbohydrate and nutrient content. The Chinese focused on the different qualities and primary actions of foods which were used to help create balance in the body. This system is known as food energetics; according to this system, all foods have specific qualities and effects on the body.

Exercise is an important factor, but it is a matter of balance: moderate exercise gets the *qi* flowing in the body but excessive amounts drain our vital kidney energy and can weaken the body. Understanding the concepts of duality and of balancing rest with activity is essential. According to TCM, too much sex can weaken the body thus reducing our vitality and energy levels. This is explained in greater depth under the chapter on the kidney (*page 149*).

## body clock

Every organ in the body has a two-hour period of maximum activity which means that when the organ is in its natural time period, it has greater energy than the others. If we honoured these times and let them guide us in our activities we would be much healthier. If you find that you have a dip in energy or feel worse at a particular time of day, then this could be pointing to the particular organ which falls into that time period. For example, the stomach is in power between 7 and 9 a.m. This is the time that digestion is at its peak. Therefore, the old advice 'Breakfast like a

King, lunch like a Prince and dine like a Pauper' is in fact quite correct, as breakfast is the time of the day when the body digests foods best. If you feel particularly tired between 5 and 7 p.m. in the evening, your kidney energy may not be as strong as it should be. If you can't get to sleep between the hours of 11 p.m. and 3 a.m., then your Wood Element is out of balance and needs treatment.

## early signs of disease

The wonder of the Chinese system of medicine is that changes often begin to occur approximately six to nine months *before* a disease arises. We can pick up on the particular stress signals that nature is providing if we can understand more about the body and know what signs to look out for. The body can show imbalances in a variety of ways: a hatred or passion for a particular season of the year, a love of a particular colour or a desire to avoid wearing a specific colour, or even a change in the colour of your face. Your body will emit a specific odour when an organ becomes imbalanced, and your emotions will change (since the organs in the body influence our emotions). By understanding and listening to your body, you can find out why it is functioning the way it is and then take the necessary steps towards improving your health.

The table below charts the traditional Chinese interpretations given to each of the five elements and its related organs.

## five elements table

|  | Wood | Fire | Earth | Metal | Water |
|---|---|---|---|---|---|
| Direction | East | South | Centre | West | North |
| Colour | Green | Red | Yellow | White | Blue/Black |
| Climate | Wind | Heat | Humidity | Dryness | Cold |
| Season | Spring | Summer | Late Summer | Autumn | Winter |
| Yin Organ | Liver | Heart | Spleen | Lungs | Kidneys |
| Time | 1–3 a.m. | 11a.m.–1 p.m. | 9–11 a.m. | 3–5 a.m. | 5–7 p.m. |
| Yang Organ | Gall Bladder | Small Intestine | Stomach | Large Intestine | Bladder |
| Time | 11 p.m.–1 a.m. | 1–3 p.m. | 7–9 a.m. | 5–7a.m. | 3–5 p.m. |
| Stage | Birth | Growth | Transformation | Absorption | Storage |
| Number | 8 | 7 | 5 | 9 | 6 |
| Planet | Jupiter | Mars | Saturn | Venus | Mercury |
| Spirit | Hun | Shen | Yi | P'o | Zhi |
| Body Tissue | Tendons/ Ligaments | Blood Vessels | Muscles/Flesh | Skin | Bones/ Marrow |
| Voice Sound | Shouting | Laughter | Singing | Weeping | Moaning |
| Emotion | Anger | Joy | Worry/ Sympathy | Grief | Fear |
| Taste | Sour | Bitter | Sweet | Spicy | Salty |
| Odour | Rancid | Burnt | Fragrant | Pungent | Putrid |
| Sense Organ | Eyes | Tongue | Mouth | Nose | Ears |
| Reflector | Nails | Complexion | Lips | Body Hair | Head Hair |
| Secretion | Tears | Perspiration | Saliva | Nasal Discharge | Sputum |

**N.B.** The time for the *pericardium* is 7–9 p.m.; for the *triple warmer*, 9–11 p.m.

# creating a naturally better future

Despite the differences between conventional and natural medicine, both Eastern and Western approaches have their value for the sick patient. So often we take for granted that Western methods are the best, but the ancient wisdom of the East can make an equally important contribution; an optimal approach to future healthcare should be a combined approach? Natural medicine and traditional healing methods are undoubtedly excellent long-term approaches to maintaining health, as they are gentle yet highly effective. However, conventional medicine is appropriate in certain situations including life-threatening emergencies and those that require surgery. Eastern and Western methods should become more integrated in the next decade as we move towards a truly eclectic medical system where the chief objective should be to restore balance, harmonious function and wellbeing.

The notion of healing yourself is at the root of the natural and Chinese Medicine philosophy. As more individuals have witnessed first-hand the harmful effects that occur due to the over-use or misuse of modern medical drugs, they are turning to gentler, less invasive techniques that do not have such a disruptive effect on the body and which invoke self-healing. We need to recognize that the individual can play a fundamental role in his or her own healing process.

In today's society, we have forgotten how to create the right conditions for the body to heal itself. Factors such as inappropriate lifestyle, poor diet and the polluted environment we have created, all abuse the delicate working systems of our body. For millions of years, man has been eating a simple diet of unrefined, organic produce, yet in this century we have resorted to using technology and chemicals to process, and consequently adulterate, our food. I urge you all to start supporting the organic movement and purchasing as many items as possible that are organic. I do realize that the costs are higher, however, if more of us support organic farming by putting our hands in our pockets and purchasing the produce, then prices will lower. Remember that when we eat organic food, that is simply food grown without the use of harmful chemicals and pesticides, you will not only be providing your body with a richer source of vitamins and minerals, but you will be supporting the earth you live on. The pesticides that are sprayed on to crops make their way into the air we breathe, the food we eat and the water we drink. So sadly, even when we eat organic foods environmental pollutants and toxins are still affecting us. This is why I am stressing so much to you the importance of supporting the organic movement for our future and the future of our planet. I believe it is now time for us all to take responsibility for our precious Mother Earth who sustains, nurtures and supports us with food, water and healing plants. We should never take her gifts for granted, rather we should respect her and give thanks for all that she supplies. We should nurture her in the same way that we should nurture ourselves.

When you develop compassion, love and respect for your body, emotions and soul, you will want to take more care of it. When you can visibly and tangibly feel the positive changes that occur when you begin to get your body back into balance, you will intuitively start to choose things in your life that support and nourish you rather than weaken you. I can merely guide you and awaken your desire to make these changes – give you the instruction manual helping you to navigate your own personal course to health and wellbeing. NOW IS THE TIME. There comes a point when you simply have to understand that the decision to make changes lies within you and only you ... the wisdom lies within. However, adopting a new approach and creating meaningful lifestyle changes is a major undertaking that requires both effort and dedication. With the hectic pace of life that we all lead, it is easy to procrastinate. But at some point in our life it is important to look past the long list of reasons not to change, and realize what can be gained by making a commitment to a better way of life. Time moves on and with each new day we are either a day nearer our goal or a day further away.

The rewards of having a finely tuned, firm, strong healthy body far outweigh the initial sacrifices you will have to make on the road to change. You will possess a serenity of spirit, an ability to cope, react and adapt to the stressful times of the new millennium, attain a level of peace and tranquillity that you never thought possible, have an inner radiance, glow and beauty that no amount of expensive face creams or cosmetic surgery could ever give you and a love and respect of the body you inhabit and the life that you lead. This life, your life, is all about honouring and being at one with your own body, the only one you will ever have in this lifetime. I truly wish you health and happiness on your journey through life and hope that you will find your own wisdom within.

creating a naturally better future

# healing recipes

With all of the recipes, wherever possible choose organic produce. The quantities in the recipes are flexible – I am the sort of cook who never measures anything, but throws in whatever is there … so do feel free to experiment and be creative with these dishes!

## stomach

### SUNSHINE BREAKFAST

Some of you may frown when you see that eggs are the main ingredients for the stomach recipe. However, as the stomach is in power between 7 and 9 a.m. – breakfast time, then it is an ideal time for the hydrochloric acid in the stomach to break down proteins. The cayenne pepper aids digestion and has a reputation of helping to heal stomach ulcers if used in small amounts. The rice cheese is a delicious alternative to dairy cheese (which I find indigestible when cooked) and goes all gooey and adds to the wonderful golden yellow colour of the dish, golden yellow being the colour for the Earth Element. I have not recommended that you eat this with a carbohydrate such as toast, for those individuals who wish to food combine.

2 large eggs, beaten with a little water added
2 fresh chopped tomatoes
2 slices of American Rice cheese (Galaxy Foods)
sprinkle of cayenne pepper
handful of chopped fresh herbs to taste (basil, coriander etc)
1 teaspoon of olive oil

1  Heat the oil in a frying pan and add the cayenne pepper. Add to this the chopped tomatoes and stir-fry for about a minute.
2  Add the beaten eggs ensuring that the base of the pan is totally covered.
3  Slice the rice cheese into thin strips and lay across the top of the eggs while they cook.
4  Sprinkle on fresh herbs and when the omelette is cooked, fold in half and serve.

## spleen

### MEDITERRANEAN TOFU BAKE

Yams and carrots, rich in beta carotene, are excellent root vegetables for the spleen and being cooked in apple juice, together with the natural sweetness of apricot (the fruit for the Earth Element) all help to nourish the spleen. The spleen does need warm food in preference to raw and the good news is that although some vitamin C is lost during cooking, one study has shown that beta carotene is absorbed more effectively when vegetables are cooked! Tofu is a valuable source of calcium and is dairy-free. However, it has a cold energy so is best either marinated in ginger prior to cooking, or as with this dish, include plenty of ginger.

1 large yam, cut into cubes
1 large red and yellow pepper cut into cubes
1 punnet cherry tomatoes, cut in half
6 apricots
2 medium carrots, cut into thin strips
2 scallions (spring onions)
1 pack tofu, 250g cut in slices
1 large piece of ginger, grated
pinch of cayenne and black pepper
1 glass of pure apple juice
1 tablespoon of sesame oil

1   Put 2 tablespoons of apple juice into a pan and sweat the scallions, yam, peppers, carrots and ginger until they begin to soften.
2   Add the remaining apple juice and tomatoes and bake covered in the oven at a moderate temperature for 20 minutes, until yam is tender.
3   Lay slices of tofu on top of the vegetable mix, drizzle sesame oil over tofu and sprinkle on a pinch of cayenne pepper and sesame seeds.
4   Put under a hot grill until toasted and serve with coriander millet.
5   If you want to food combine, then omit the tofu from the recipe, making the meal a carbohydrate based meal.


**CORIANDER MILLET**

Millet as we know, nourishes the spleen and the warming energy of coriander seeds are excellent for acute indigestion, bloating and gas as well as being a good energy tonic. The fresh leaves have weaker and cooler properties but are packed with vitamins and minerals.

100g millet
600ml water
Fresh and dried coriander

1  Wash and cook the millet in the boiling water until just tender and all the water has been absorbed. Do not over-cook, otherwise you will find yourself with a lump of sticky stodge!

2  Mix in the fresh coriander and black pepper. I sometimes gently heat a little oil and add some ground coriander to this – cook for a minute and then add the millet. Fresh coriander can then be added before serving.

## heart

### HEARTY MACKEREL

In Japan, the incidence of heart disease is statistically much lower; this has been scientifically linked to their diet which is very low in saturated fats and high in fish. A Dutch study showed that if each person ate only 25g of oily fish per day it would cut the chances of fatal heart attack by half. Olive oil is used liberally in cooking in the Mediterranean areas and they have a very low incidence of heart disease.

2 mackerel (cleaned)
1 red onion
2 lemons
2 large tomatoes
2 large garlic cloves and a handful of parsley
1 slice wholemeal bread
3-4 tablespoons virgin olive oil
1 tablespoon runny honey and 1 tablespoon of tamari sauce

1  Put garlic, parsley and the slice of bread (can be wheat-free alternative such as rye) into a blender and when it is a fine crumb texture, add olive oil to give you a crumble mixture.

2  Slit the mackerel diagonally almost to the bone 3 times and stuff the slits with the breadcrumb mixture.

3    Cover the mackerel with a slice of lemon followed by a slice of tomato until the fish is covered.

4    Lay the sliced onion on top and drizzle with olive oil. To add extra flavour, you can add tamari sauce and honey which can also be drizzled on to the fish.

5    Bake in a medium hot oven for 15 minutes until the fish comes easily off the bone.

6    Add extra parsley to garnish (and counteract the garlic).

7    Serve with a salad of fresh bitter greens such as radicchio, rocket, bitter endive, chicory and dandelion.

8    For the dressing, use 2 tablespoons of an Essential fatty acid oil mix such as Udo's Choice with either cider or balsamic vinegar, lemon juice and include fresh garden herbs and crushed garlic. Shake well in a jar and pour over the salad. (*See recipe page 287*)


## small intestine

### SALMON AND CARROT FISH CAKES WITH YOGHURT DIP

This is a terribly healthy and delicious recipe that I made by accident one day when I was trying to decide what to do with the pulp from my carrot juice. Its orange colour is energizing to the small intestine, it is wheat and dairy free (if you use a soya-based yoghurt for the dip) and follows the principles of food combining too. If you do not wish to adhere to this, you can probably make a much tastier version using mashed potato! There is lots of fibre in the carrot pulp, calcium and fatty acids in the tinned salmon and when combined with all the acidophilus contained in the natural yoghurt makes it an ideal recipe for your small intestine!

Pulp from 8 carrots and a piece of ginger left over from juicing
400g canned salmon
Handful of the fine dry seaweed (wakame)
Large handful of fresh chopped herbs such as basil and tarragon

2 eggs

1 small tub natural yoghurt (can be soya, sheep or goat's milk)

2 cloves garlic

4 tablespoons buckwheat flour (optional crushed coriander seeds)

3 tablespoons virgin olive oil

1   Squeeze excess water out of your carrot pulp (left over from juicing fresh carrots and ginger).

2   Strain salmon and combine with the carrot pulp, the dried seaweed (which helps to absorb excess water) together with half of the chopped, fresh herbs and make into patties.

3   Beat the eggs and dip the patties into the mix – this is the incredibly messy bit as the patties often crumble as they do not have much to bind them, so you have to be quite forceful! If you are concerned about your cholesterol, you can use the egg whites to bind but I prefer to use the whole egg.

4   Lightly dust the patties with a fine layer of buckwheat flour and heat a pan with your olive oil. If you suffer from intestinal spasms and wind, you can mix a teaspoon of ground coriander in with the flour to aid digestion. To make less mess, you can line a loaf tin with a smear of olive oil and bake in an oven rather like a nut loaf.

5   Place the patties in the oil over a medium heat and cook for approximately 15 minutes, turning when golden brown, ensuring that they are cooked inside.

6   Crush the garlic and add to the yoghurt with the other half of your fresh garden herbs. Stir well and serve to accompany the fish cakes.

## bladder

### COLOURFUL CRANBERRY AND CARROT SOUP

I was once recommending cranberries to a patient who was suffering from cystitis and advising her not to purchase cranberry juice with a high sugar content. Contemplating the thought of how cranberry needed natural sweetness, I then devised this recipe that combines the sweetness of carrots to counteract the sharpness of the cranberries. An onion is included as this is a natural food cure for urinary tract infections. I also added spices such as nutmeg and cinnamon to give the Water Element that extra warmth it so often needs.

450g carrots, chopped
1 punnet of cranberries
1 large red onion
500ml cranberry and apple juice and 500ml vegetable stock
Sprinkling of grated nutmeg and cinnamon

1 Sweat the onion in a little of the cranberry and apple juice (or use a splash of boiling water) and add the carrots.
2 Then add your cranberries and extra water or juice and cook over a low heat for about 10 minutes, until carrots are tender. Allow to cool.
3 Put into a food processor and blend into a purée. The consistency is very much up to personal taste – you can add more liquid accordingly.
4 Add grated nutmeg and ground cinnamon to taste.

## kidney

### SALMON AND KIDNEY BEANS DISH

The night before a breakfast television programme, I was suddenly phoned by the producer and asked to bring a dish in that would be a quick and easy dish, ideal for the Winter. Shops were closed at this time, so I had to put my thinking cap on. I raided my larder and pulled out my ever favourite Ready Rice by Whole Earth which is organic pre-cooked rice which is a godsend when you can't wait 40 minutes for brown rice to cook! My next favourite, tinned wild red Alaskan salmon, followed by a can of kidney beans. So this is my healthy 'convenience' food dish which takes no longer than 5 minutes to prepare! It also contains seaweed, excellent for the kidneys, garlic for its vasodilatory action to increase the circulation and warm our cold bodies in the Winter months, turmeric, another spice known for its warming action on the body. Parsley, an excellent diuretic, completes the dish as a garnish.

440g can of Ready Rice (Whole Earth)
440g can wild red salmon
440g kidney beans
Generous handful of dried seaweed strips (wakame)
2 tablespoons virgin olive oil
2 cloves crushed garlic, 1 teaspoon turmeric and cayenne pepper to taste
Parsley to garnish

1  Take the tiny shredded pieces of seaweed and soak in water.
2  Gently heat the oil and add the crushed garlic, turmeric and cayenne pepper. Cook for one minute on low heat.
3  Add the rice and ensure that it is thoroughly mixed with the spices.
4  Drain the kidney beans, salmon and seaweed and then add to the rice.
5  Gently heat the entire mix until hot and serve with parsley sprinkled on top.

## liver and gall bladder

### KICHAREE AND A BITTER GREEN SALAD

So often today, the trend is to go on a short fruit fast to detoxify your body. However, this does indeed put great pressure on the organs of elimination, which are already under considerable strain due to the toxins in the air we breath, water we drink and food we eat. Gentle detoxification is the key as then we prepare the body to eliminate toxins from a deeper level (liver, kidney etc), so giving the superficial organs of elimination such as the bowels time to adjust and release effectively. Kicharee is viewed as a healing recipe that has been used in Indian medicine as a fasting meal as it was considered to slowly cleanse the body and bring about balance to both *yin* and *yang*. I have served it here with a bitter salad with the essential fatty acids to enhance gall bladder function.

> 1 cup of mung beans
> 1 can of Ready Rice
> 3 teaspoons olive oil
> 1 teaspoon of turmeric, cumin and coriander

1  Soak the beans overnight and wash thoroughly.
2  Cook the mung beans for 40 minutes in boiling water until slightly soft. Drain.
3  Add spices to the olive oil and gently cook for a few minutes to release their flavour.
4  Add the Ready Rice and mung beans, coating the beans and rice with the spices.
5  When mixture is hot, serve with a salad of fresh bitter greens such as radicchio, rocket, bitter endive, chicory and dandelion.
6  For the dressing, use 3 tablespoons of Udo's Choice Essential fatty acid oil mix (to support liver and gall bladder function) with either 1 tablespoon of organic cider or balsamic vinegar or the juice of a lemon. Add 1 teaspoon honey, ½ teaspoon of mustard, 1 teaspoon freshly grated ginger and 1 clove freshly crushed garlic. Shake well in a jar and pour over the salad. Store the remainder in the fridge and use in a few days.

# lungs

## SPICY SOUP

This is a wonderfully colourful and warming soup that contains many foods that support lung function including garlic, thyme, apples, apricots, walnuts, onions, cinnamon, coriander, ginger and carrots.

500g carrots, chopped
6 fresh apricots (or 12 dried which have been soaked)
1 large red onion, chopped into rings
2-3 cloves garlic, crushed
2 tablespoons freshly grated ginger
1 teaspoon ground cinnamon
1 teaspoon ground coriander and handful of fresh leaves
1 teaspoon thyme or fresh sprigs
1 tablespoon virgin olive oil
500ml water or stock
500ml apple juice
handful of chopped walnuts

1 Sweat the onion, garlic, thyme and spices on a low heat for a few minutes.
2 Add carrots and apricots and add liquid.
3 Bring to boil then cover and simmer for about 15 minutes (until carrots are tender).
4 Allow to cool and liquidize until smooth.
5 Serve sprinkled with fresh coriander and chopped walnuts.

# large intestine

## LUSCIOUS VEGGIES

This is a simple vegetable dish which is a light healthy meal, and is actually rather filling too! High in a gentle form of fibre that is not taxing to your body to process that can help to clear your colon and is rich in vitamins, minerals and essential fatty acids to lubricate your intestines due to the addition of the Udo's choice oil. This is for one person, and you can select vegetables according to the season and what is available locally. Fresh herbs such as basil (ideal for constipation) can be sprinkled on prior to serving.

2 large pieces of curly dark green kale, shredded
1 large carrot, chopped into fine sticks
1 large courgette (zucchini) cut into fine rings
8 cherry tomatoes
2 slices mozzarella rice cheese or rice parmesan (Galaxy Foods)
2 tablespoons of Udo's Choice organic oil
Fresh herbs such as basil and garlic

1 Put all the vegetables except the tomatoes into a steamer and cook for 5 minutes (according to personal preference) and then add the tomatoes and cook for another 2 minutes.

2 If you would like to include garlic, I crush 2 cloves and mix them in with the essential fatty acids oil, drizzle on the vegetables and sprinkle with rice parmesan, or strips of mozzarella rice cheese and fresh basil.

# useful addresses

**General Council and Register of Naturopaths**
Goswell House
Goswell Road
Street
Somerset BA16 0JG
UK Tel: +44 (0)1458 840072

**The Complementary Medicine Association**
142 Greenwich High Road
London SE10 8NN
UK Tel: +44 (0)20 8305 9571
www.the-cma.org.uk

**British Complementary Medicine Association**
35 Prestbury Road
Cheltenham
Glos GS5Q 2PT
UK Tel: +44 (0)1242 519911

**British Holistic Medical Association**

Trust House

Royal Shrewsbury Hospital South

Shrewsbury SY3 8XF

UK  Tel: +44 (0)1743 261155


**The Natural Medicines Society**

PO Box 232

East Molesey

Surrey KT9 1BW

UK  Tel: +44 (0)20 8224 0200


**Institute for Complementary Medicine**

PO Box 194

London SE16 1QZ

UK  Tel: +44 (0)20 7237 5165

(Please send an SAE with two first class stamps)


**What The Doctors Don't Tell You**

77 Grosvenor Avenue

London N5 2NN

UK  Tel: +44 (0)20 7354 4592 or +44 (0)800 146054

www.wddty.co.uk

(They have a range of valuable handbooks on subjects such as cancer,

vaccinations, women's screenings etc.)


**Friends of the Earth**

26-28 Underwood Street

London N1 7JQ

UK  Tel: +44 (0)20 7490 1555 or +44 (0)990 224 488

www.foe.co.uk

**Greenpeace**

Canonbury Villas

London N1 2PN

UK Tel: +44 (0)20 7865 8100

(www.truefood.org)

**Jennifer Harper**

PO Box 150

Woking

Surrey GU23 6XS

UK

www.jenniferharper.com

**School of Complementary Studies**

University of Westminster

35 Marylebone Road

London NW1 5LS

UK Tel: +44 (0)20 7911 5082

www. wmin. ac. uk

## AROMATHERAPY & NATURAL BODYCARE

**The Aromatherapy Organisations Council**

PO Box 19834

London SE25 6WF

UK Tel: +44 (0)20 8251 7912

**International Federation of Aromatherapists**

Stamford House

2–4 Chiswick High Road

London W4 1TH

UK Tel: +44 (0)20 8742 2605

**The International Society of Professional Aromatherapists**
82 Ashby Road
Hinkley
Leics LE10 1SN
UK  Tel: +44 (0)1455 637987

**Dr Hauschka UK**
19-20 Stockwood Business Park
Stockwood
Near Redditch
Worcestershire B96 6SX
UK  Tel: +44 (0)1386 792622

**Dr Hauschka Cosmetics USA Inc**
59C North Street
Hatfield, MA 01038
USA
Tel: +1 800 247 9907

**Aveda Ltd**
7 Munton Road
London SE17 1PR
UK  Tel: +44 (0)20 7410 1600

**Aveda Corporation (US)**
4000 Pheasant Ridge Drive
Blaine
MN 55449-7106
USA Tel: +1 612 783 4000
www.aveda.com

**The Green People Company Ltd**

Brighton Road

Handcross

West Sussex RH17 6B2

UK  Tel: +44 (0)1444 401444

www.greenpeople.co.uk

**Origins (UK)**

73 Grosvenor Street

London W1X 0BH

UK  Tel: +44 (0)800 731 4039

www.origins.com


**Origins (US)**

757 5th Avenue

New York, NY 10153

USA

Tel: +1 800 ORIGINS

www.origins.com


## CHINESE MEDICINE

**British Acupuncture Council**

206–208 Latimer Road

London W10 6RE

UK  Tel: +44 (0)20 8964 0222


**Register of Chinese Herbal Medicine**

PO Box 400

Wembley

Middlesex HA9 9NZ

UK  Tel: +44 (0)20 7224 0883 or 0)20 8904 1357

## CHIROPRACTORS

**McTimoney Chiropractic Association**
21 High Street

Eynsham
Oxfordshire OX8 1HE
UK Tel: +44 (0)1865 880974


## CRANIOSACRAL THERAPY

**Craniosacral Therapy Association of the UK**
27 Old Gloucester Street
London WC1N 3XX
UK Tel: +44 (0)7000 784735


## FLOWER REMEDIES

**Dr Edward Bach Foundation**
Mount Vernon
Sotwell
Wallingford OX10 0PZ
UK Tel: +44 (0)20 8780 4200

**Healing Herbs' Bach Flower Remedies**
PO Box 65
Hereford HR2 0UW
UK Tel: +44 (0)1873 890218

**Institute of Phytobiophysics**

10 St James Street

St Helier

Jersey JE2 3QZ

UK  Tel: +44 (0)1534 738737

www.phytobiophysics.com

**International Flower Essence Repertoire**

The Living Tree

Milland

Liphook

Hants GU3 7JS

UK  Tel: +44 (0)1428 741572

Email: flower@atlas.co.uk


## HERBS & SUPPLEMENTS

**Schoenenberger Plant Juices (UK)**

Phyto Products Limited

Park Works

Park Road

Mansfield Woodhouse

Nottinghamshire NG19 8EF

UK  Tel: +44 (0)1623 644334 and Fax:+44 (0)1623 657232


**Schoenenberger Plant Juices (US)**

Bio-Nutritional Products

PO Box 9

Harrington Park

NY 07640

USA

**Udo's Choice Oil (UK)**
Savant Distribution
15 Iveson Approach
Leeds LS16 6LJ
UK  Tel: +44 (0)113 230 1993
www.savant-health.com

**Udo's Choice Oil (US)**
Flora Inc.
805 East Badger Road
Lynden, WA 98264
USA
Tel: +1 360 354 2110
www.florahealth.com

**Solgar Corporate World Headquarters**
500 Frank W Boulevard
Teaneck
New Jersey NJ 07666
USA
Tel: +1 201 944 2311
www.solgar.com

**Solgar Vitamins (UK)**
Aldbury
Tring
Herts HP23 5PT
UK Tel: +44 (0)1442 890355

**National Institute of Medical Herbalists**
56 Longbrook Street
Exeter EX4 6AH
UK Tel: +44 (0)1392  426022

**Unified Register of Herbal Practitioners**

PO Box 126

Crowborough TN7 4ZR

UK Tel: +44 (0) 1303 814816

**Klamath Blue Green Algae**

PO Box 1626

Mount Shasta

California 96067

USA  Tel: +1 800 327 1956

www.klamathbluegreen.com

**Klamath Blue Green Algae**

The Really Healthy Company Ltd

PO Box 4390

London SW15 6YQ

UK  Tel/fax:  +44 (0)20 8780 5200

**Biocare**

Lakeside

180 Lifford Lane

Kings Norton B30 3NU

UK  Tel: +44 (0)121 433 3727

## MAIL ORDER HERBS & SUPPLEMENTS

**The Nutri-Centre**

The Hale Clinic

7 Park Crescent

London W1N 3HE

UK  Tel: +44 (0)20 7436 5122

E-mail: enq@nutricentre.com

**Hambleden Herbs (organic herbs)**
Court Farm
Milverton
Somerset TA4 1NF
UK Tel: +44 (0)1823 401205
www.hambledenherbs.co.uk

**Farmacia**
169 Drury Lane
Covent Garden
London WC2B 5QA
UK Tel: +44 (0)20 7831 0830
www.farmacia.co.uk

**Healing Herb Supplies (Organic Herbs)**
5 Popes Cross
Curry Mallet
Taunton
Somerset TA3 6SS
UK  Tel: +44 (0)1823 481193


**HOMOEOPATHY**

**The Society of Homoeopaths**
2 Artisan Road
Northampton NN1 4HU
UK  Tel: +44 (0)1604  621400

**The UK Homoeopathic Medical Association**
6 Livingstone Road
Gravesend
Kent DA12 5DZ
UK  Tel: +44 (0)1474 560336

## ORGANIC PRODUCE

**Henry Doubleday Research Association**
Ryton Organic Gardens
Ryton-on-Dunsmor
Coventry CV8 3LG
UK  Tel: +44 (0)2476 303 517
Email: enquiry@hdra.org.uk

**Pipers Farm (organic meat)**
Peter and Henrietta Greig
Pipers Farm
Cullompton
Devon EX15 1SD
UK  Tel: +44 (0)1392 881380 Fax: +44 (0)1392 881600

**Galaxy Foods Rice Slices** – distributed in UK by
Brewhurst Health Food Supplies Limited
Abbot Close
Byfleet
Surrey KT14 7JP
UK  Tel: +44 (0)1932 354211

**Planet Organic**
42 Westbourne Grove
London W2 5SH
UK  Tel: +44 (0)20 7221 7171

**The Soil Association**
86 Colston Street
Bristol BS1 5BB
UK  Tel: +44 (0)117 929 0661

**Wild Oats**
210 Westbourne Grove
London
W11 2RH
UK  Tel: +44 (0)20 7229 1063

**Freshlands**
49 Parkway
London NW1 7PN
UK  Tel: +44 (0)20 7428 7575
(also at 196 Old Street, London)

**Infinity Foods**
25 North Road
Brighton
East Sussex BN1 1YA
UK  Tel: +44 (0)1273 603 563

**PSYCHOTHERAPY**

**The National Council of Psychotherapists**
Head Office
Hazelwood
Broadmead
Sway
Hants SO41 6DH
UK  Tel: +44 (0)1590 683770

## NUTRITION AND HEALING

**British Association of Nutritional Therapists**
PO Box 17436
London SE13 7WT
UK  Tel: +44 (0)870 606 1284

**National Federation of Spiritual Healers**
Old Manor Farm Studio
Church Street
Sunbury-on-Thames
Middlesex TW16 6RG
UK  Tel: +44 (0)1932 783164  Healer referral line: +44 (0)891 616080

**The Institute for Optimum Nutrition**
Blades Court
Deodar Road
London SW15 2NU
UK  Tel: +44 (0)20 8877 9993

**Society for the Promotion of Nutritional Therapy**
PO Box 47
Heathfield
East Sussex TN21 8ZX
UK  Tel: +44 (0)1825 872921

## REFLEXOLOGY

**Association of Reflexologists**
27 Old Gloucester Street
London WC1N 3XX
UK  Tel: +44 (0)990 673320

# suggested reading

Bateson-Koch DC ND, Carolee. *Allergies: Disease in Disguise*, Alive Books, 1998

Brecher, Paul. *Principles of Tai Chi*, Thorsons, 1997

Chopra MD, Deepak. *The Seven Spiritual Laws of Success*, Bantam Press, 1996

—, *Ageless Body, Timeless Mind*, Rider, 1998

—, *Boundless Energy*, Rider, 1995

Clark, Susan. *The Sunday Times Vitality Cookbook*, HarperCollins, 1999

Courtenay, Hazel and Briffa, John. *What's the Alternative?*, Boxtree, 1996

Devereux, Godfrey. *Dynamic Yoga*, Thorsons, 1998

Eden, Donna. *Energy Medicine*, Piatkus, 1999

Erasmus, Udo. *Fats that Heal, Fats that Kill*, Alive Books, 1999

Geddes, Nicola and Lockie, Dr Andrew. *Women's Guide to Homeopathy*, Hamish Hamilton, 1993

Gursche MH, Siegfried and Rona MD MSc, Zoltan. *Encyclopedia of Natural Healing*, Alive Books, 1998

Hicks, Angela. *The Five Laws for Healthy Living*, Thorsons, 1998

Jones, Hilary. *Doctor What's the Alternative*, Coronet, 1999

Kenton, Leslie. *Journey to Freedom*, HarperCollins, 1998

—, *Passage to Power* Vermilion, 1996

Linford, Monica. *Awaken Your Body, Balance Your Mind,* Thorsons, 2000

Lockie, Dr Andrew. *The Family Guide to Homeopathy*, Hamish Hamilton, 1998

Manning, Matthew. *One Foot in the Stars*, Element, 1999

—, *No Faith Required*, Eikstein, 1995

McTaggart, Lynne. *What Doctors Don't Tell You*, Thorsons, 1996

Myss PhD, Caroline. *Anatomy of the Spirit*, Bantam, 1997

—, *The Creation of Health,* Bantam, 1999

—, *Why People Don't Heal and How They Can*, Bantam, 1998

Peters, David. *Total Health*, Marshall Publishing, 1998

Rechelbacher, Horst. *Aveda Rituals*, Ebury Press, 1999

Smyth, Angela and Jones, Dr Hilary. *The Complete Encyclopaedia of Natural Health*, Thorsons, 1997

Stengler ND, Mark. *The Natural Physician*, Alive Books, 1997

de Vries, Jan. *Inner Harmony,* Mainstream Publishing Company, 1999

—, *How to Lead a Healthy Life*, Mainstream Publishing Company, 1995

Woodham, Anne and Peters, Dr David. *The Encyclopedia of Complementary Medicine*, Dorling Kindersley, 1997

## AROMATHERAPY

Davis, Patricia. *Aromatherapy: an A–Z*, C. W. Daniel, 1995

Hopkins, Cathy. *Principles of Aromatherapy*, Thorsons, 1996

Lawless, Julia. *Aromatherapy and the Mind*, Thorsons, 1998

Mojay, Gabriel. *Aromatherapy for Healing the Spirit*, Gaia Books, 1996

Price, Shirley. *Practical Aromatherapy*, Thorsons, 1994

— *Aromatherapy Workbook: understanding essential oils*, Thorsons, 1993

Sellar, Wanda. *The Directory of Essential Oils*, C. W. Daniel, 1992

Worwood, Valerie Ann. *The Fragrant Pharmacy: a complete guide to aromatherapy and essential oils*, Bantam Books, 1991

## CHINESE MEDICINE

Chang, Dr Stephen. *The Complete System of Chinese Self-Healing*, Thorsons, 1998

Chia, Mantak and Maneewan. *Chi Nei Tsang: internal organs chi massage*, Healing Tao Books, 1991

Connelly, Dianne M. *Traditional Acupuncture: the law of the five elements*, Traditional Acupuncture Institute, 1994

Gach, Michael Reed. *Acupressure: how to cure common ailments the natural way*, Piatkus Books, 1993

Hicks, Angela. *Principles of Chinese Medicine*, Thorsons, 1996

Kaptchuk, Ted J. *Chinese Medicine: the web has no weaver*, Century Paperbacks, 1987

Teeguarden, Iona Marsaa. *Acupressure Way of Health: Jin Shin Do*, Japan Publications, 1978

Tierra, Lesley. *Herbs of Life: health and healing using Western and Chinese techniques*, Crossing Press, 1992

Williams PhD, Tom. *Chinese Medicine: Acupuncture, Herbal Remedies, Nutrition, Qigong and Health Essentials*, Element Books, 1995

Young, Jacqueline. *Acupressure for Health: a complete self-care manual*, Thorsons, 1994

—, *Acupressure Step by Step*, Thorsons, 1998

## FLOWER REMEDIES

Ball, Stefan. *Principles of Bach Flower Remedies*, Thorsons, 1999

Kramer & Wild, *New Bach Flower Body Maps*, Healing Arts Press, 1996

Scheffer, Mechthild. *Bach Flower Therapy: theory and practice*, Thorsons, 1986

## HERBALISM

Gursche, Siegfried. *Healing with Herbal Juices*, Alive Books, 1993

Hoffman, David. *Thorsons Guide to Medical Herbalism*, Thorsons, 1991

Mills, Simon. *The Complete Guide to Modern Herbalism*, Thorsons, 1994

Tierra, Michael. *Planetary Herbology*, Lotus Light Publications, 1989

de Vries, Jan. By Appointment Only series, Mainstream Publishing Company, 1995

Dr Vogel, H. C. A. *Nature Doctor: manual of traditional medicine*, Mainstream
  Publishing Company, 1990

## NUTRITION AND HEALING

Abrams, Korl J. *Algae to the Rescue*, Logan House Publications, 1996

Andrea, Judith. *Wheels of Life*, Llewellyn Publications, 1998

Brewer, Dr Sarah. *Candida Albicans*, Thorsons, 1997

Carper, Jean. *Miracle Cures*, Thorsons, 1997

—, *Stop Ageing Now*, Thorsons, 1997

Chaitow ND DO, Leon. *The Antibiotic Crisis: Antibiotic Alternatives*, Thorsons,
  1998

Chopra MD, Deepak. *Perfect Health*, Bantam, 1990

Courtenay, Hazel. *Divine Intervention*, Cima Books, 1999

D'Adamo, Dr Peter J. and Catherine Whitney. *Eat Right For Your Type*, Putnam,
  1997

Grant, Doris and Joice, Jean. *Food Combining for Health*, Thorsons, 1991

Haas MD, Elson M. *Staying Healthy with Nutrition*, Celestial Arts, 1992

Holford, Patrick. *100% Health*, Piatkus, 1999

—, *The Optimum Nutrition Bible*, Piatkus Books, 1998

Holford, Patrick and Ridgway, Judy. *The Optimum Nutrition Cookbook*, Piatkus,
  1999

Kenton, Leslie. *Lean Revolution*, Ebury Press, 1994

—, *10 Day De-Stress Plan*, Ebury Press, 1994

—, *10 Steps to Energy*, Ebury Press, 1997

Hay, Louise L. *Heal Your Body: the mental causes for physical illness*, Eden Grove
  Editions, 1989

Lazarides, Linda. *Principles of Nutritional Therapy*, Thorsons, 1996

Lidolt, Erwina. *The Food Combining Cookbook: recipes for the Hay system*,
  Thorsons, 1993

Lu, Henry C. *Chinese System of Food Cures: prevention and remedies*, USA, Sterling Publications, 1986

Marsden, Kathryn. *The Food Combining Diet: lose weight and stay healthy with the Hay system*, Thorsons, 1993

Matthews, Andrew. *Being Happy*, Media Masters Masters, 1988

Northrup, Dr Christiane. *Women's Bodies, Women's Wisdom*, Piatkus, 1998

Page, Dr Christine. *Frontiers of Health: from healing to wholeness*, C. W. Daniel, 1992

—, *The Mirror of Existence: stepping into wholeness*, C. W. Daniel, 1995

Smyth, Angela, edited by Jones, Dr Hilary. *The Complete Encyclopaedia of Natural Health*, Thorsons, 1997

Van Straten, Michael. *Healing Foods*, The Ivy Press, 1997

—, *Superjuice*, Mitchell Beazley, 1999

—, *The Healthy Food Directory*, Gill & Macmillan Newleaf, 1999

Weil, Dr Andrew. *Spontaneous Healing*, Warner, 1997

—, *8 Weeks to Optimum Health*, Warner, 1998

Werbach, Dr Melvyn. *Healing through Nutrition: the natural approach to treating illnesses*, Thorsons, 1995


**REFLEXOLOGY**

Bayly, Doreen E. *Reflexology Today: the stimulation of the body's healing forces through foot massage*, Healing Arts Press, 1982

Kunz, Kevin and Barbara. *The Complete Guide to Foot Reflexology*, Thorsons, 1984

—, *Hand and Food Reflexology*, Thorsons, 1986

# other jennifer harper products

*Seasons of the Soul* – Recharge your inner self and nourish your soul with this audio CD. Drawn from ancient wisdom and spiritual insight, this CD of musical meditations is designed to resolve emotions such as grief, anger, fear, worry and lack of self-love, and allow you to re-energize and empower yourself. The meditations also teach you how to protect your soul from other people's negativity and are ideal for busy people who do not have the time to meditate.

*Orgasmic, Organic Living* – An inspirational video packed with a variety of natural life-enhancing self-help techniques, simple lifestyle changes and dietary suggestions that provides an extensive visual reference useful throughout the entire year.

Both of the above are available from:
www.jenniferharper.com

**Body Wisdom Organics** – An entirely organic range of natural products formulated by Jennifer Harper and include herbal tea mixes, essential oil blends, herbal tinctures, flower essences and spices designed to balance and strengthen your weak element. A Living Organics Superfood formula that contains a synergistic blend of living foods and minerals, energetically balanced with specific herbs, complements the range. These formulas can also be taken at the start of each season to help prevent common imbalances from developing. More information about the products can be found at www.body-wisdom-organics.com and www.livingorganics.com

Alternatively, if you would like more details on the **Body Wisdom Healing Programme** or any of the above items, you can write enclosing a stamped addressed envelope to:

Body Wisdom
PO Box 150
Woking
Surrey GU23 6XS

# index

*Note*: numbers which appear in *italic* indicate where illustrations occur.

breakfast 17–18
    recipe 279–80
breast tenderness 189, 190
breathing:
    difficulties 99, 215
    exercises 222–3, 244
bronchitis 214
bruising 188, 190

caffeine 13, 133
calming foods 94–6
calves, problems 129
Cartesian approach xvi
chewing 13, 51
chilblains 74
Chinese green tea 17
Chinese nutrition 12–20
    Earth foods 49–54, 68–73
    Fire foods 91–8, 114–16
    Metal foods 218–21, 238–43
    Water foods 131–4, 151–6
    Wood foods 175-7, 193–200
cholesterol 115, 214
circulation, poor 89, 129
cirrhosis 188
citrus fruits 17
climate:
    for bladder 128
    for Earth 9, 42, 273
    for Fire 9, 83–4, 273
    for gallbladder 172
    for heart 88
    for kidneys 147
    for large intestine 235
    for liver 189

for lungs 215
for Metal 9, 210, 273
for small intestine 111
for spleen 64
for stomach 46
for Water 9, 123–4, 273
for Wood 9, 167–8, 273
co-ordination, poor 65
coeliac's disease 110, 111
coffee 13
cold, aversion to 147
cold (principle) 262, 263
colds 28, 270
colic 47
colon:
    massage 234, 244–5
    swollen 235
colour:
    for bladder 128
    and early disease signs 8, 272
    for Earth 9, 42, 273
    facial, and early disease signs 8, 89,
     272
    for Fire 9, 84, 273
    for gallbladder 172
    for heart 88
    for kidneys 147
    for large intestine 235
    for liver 189
    for lungs 215
    for Metal 9, 210, 273
    for small intestine 111
    for spleen 64
    for stomach 46
    for Water 9, 124, 273

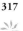

lungs/large intestine stretch 221–2, *222*

stomach/spleen stretch 54, *55*

'stuck' behaviour 67

sugar 92

Summer 2, 9, 254, 273

sunshine breakfast, recipe 279–80

Superfood Formula 16, 71

suspicion 130, 150

sweet 9, 12, 48, 273

sympathy 3, 9, 47, 67, 259, 273

symptoms of imbalance xii, 257

for bladder 129–30

for Earth 43

for Fire 85

for gallbladder 173–5

for heart 89–91

for kidneys 147–51

for large intestine 235–8

for liver 189–90

for lungs 215–17

for Metal 212

for small intestine 111–14

for spleen 65–7

for stomach 47–9

for Water 125–6

for Wood 169–70

T'ai Chi 21

taste 9, 273

for bladder 128

for gallbladder 173

for heart 88

for kidneys 147

for large intestine 235

for liver 189

for lungs 214

for small intestine 111

for spleen 65

for stomach 46

tea 13, 17, 20, 93, 94, 134, 135

tennis elbow 111

thighs, swollen and cold 65

throat, problems 111, 214, 215

thrombosis 89

thrush 173

thumb-walking technique 23

thyroid gland 6

time of day:

for bladder 128

for Earth 9, 42, 273

for Fire 9, 84, 273

for gallbladder 172

for heart 88

for kidneys 147

for large intestine 235

for liver 189

for lungs 214

for Metal 9, 210, 273

for small intestine 111

for spleen 65

for stomach 46

for Water 9, 124–5, 273

for Wood 9, 168, 273

time management 192

timidity 150

timing, of meals 8, 272

tired body 56, 65, 66

toe, stiffness 128

tongue 9, 273